Control Your IBS

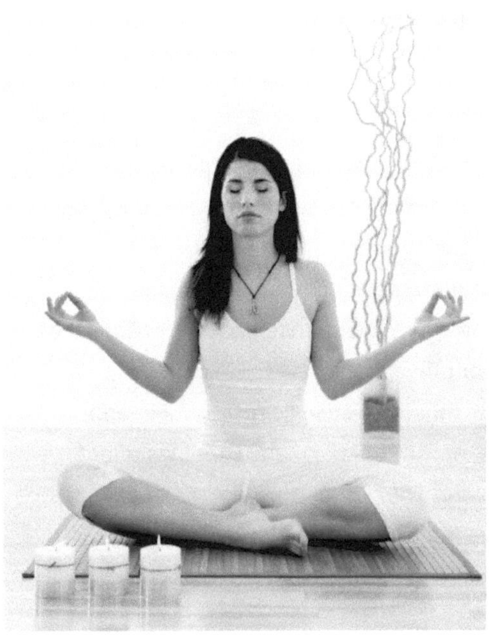

A Primer to help you understand Irritable Bowel Syndrome (IBS)

Belinda Asonganyi

ISBN: 978-0-9559809-0-9

LEGAL NOTICE

While all attempts have been made to provide effective, verifiable information in this document, neither the Author nor Publisher assumes any responsibility for errors, inaccuracies, or omissions. The information contained in this package does not make any claims or guarantees nor does it intend to provide medical advice of any kind. The information presented in this Ebook is not intended to diagnose, treat, cure, or prevent any disease. You should speak to qualified medical professional regarding specific (or even general) concerns before starting any type of exercise regime. Many variables affect each individual's results. Results will vary. The author does not make any promise of your personal success. The author has no control over what you may or may not do with this information, and therefore cannot accept the responsibility for your results.

This guide is designed for educational purposes only.

Mailto: irritabl@irritablebowel-relief.com
Website: http://www.irritablebowel-relief.com

Dedicated With Love
To Ingrid and Amy,
Without you none of this would have been worthwhile.

Awareness is to your mind what light is to a darkened room."
Peggy McColl

Table OF CONTENTS

In order to help sufferers of IBS to lead more normal lives, there are a number of lifestyle changes they can make to help reduce the uncomfortable and embarrassing symptoms of IBS. This e-book primer will give you some of the basics on this mystifying disorder and how to address the syndrome on your way back to a healthy lifestyle.

- **In Chapter 1 -** I discussed what IBS is and how the colon is supposed to work. Although IBS is not due to any structural problems with the colon or a disease, it can mimic these types of conditions. In order to rule out more serious illnesses, you will want to make plans to visit your physician's office. We also provide the roadmap for the subsequent chapters.
- **In Chapter 2 -** You will learn how you might be able to find out if you have irritable bowel syndrome. We will guide you on the many symptoms to look at and how to prepare for a visit with your physician. You will be prepared to answer the types of questions your doctor might have and thus make the most of your visit.

- **In Chapter 3 -** I will discuss the many suspects that might exacerbate IBS. Unfortunately, the medical profession still does not know what causes IBS, but they have a pretty good idea what aggravates the condition at times. Of course, this will vary from person to person, but it will help you modify your lifestyle to rule out potential triggers.

- **In Chapter 4 -** I talk about the demographics of IBS. The condition appears to manifest in late puberty or young adulthood. There are differences in gender too. In addition to this, there is some evidence that places people in industrial countries at higher risk than those in undeveloped countries. By reading who might be more likely to experience IBS, you can determine whether you are at higher risk than the average population.

- **In Chapter 5 -** I talk about a number of different approaches that can be incorporated to support your diet regimen. This gives a full approach from conventional medicines to psychotherapy and stress relief.

After reading this primer, you should be able to begin to take some steps to control this potentially devastating condition. Through diligent attention to your own lifestyle and an understanding of the options available, you can work out a plan that helps you obtain better health and happiness in your everyday life.

CHAPTER 1

WHAT IS IRRITABLE BOWEL SYNDROME?

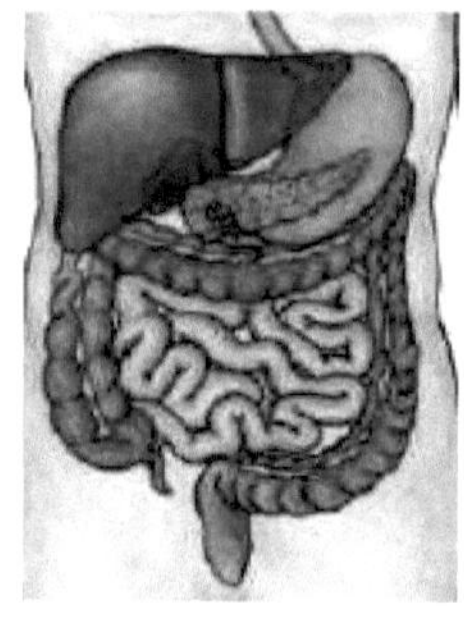

Irritable Bowel Syndrome, also known as IBS or spastic colon, is a bowel disorder that can have a number of different symptoms. Someone with IBS can have severe constipation or diarrhea or both. The condition varies from person to person in its symptoms. Other people can experience gas or abdominal pains and bloating with discomfort without any of the other symptoms. Or, they can experience a roller coaster of bowel irregularities and abdominal symptoms that can make life very difficult to manage.

The disorder often takes a while to diagnose since it will appear to have no apparent cause that can be causing the problem. There is no medical test that specifically targets IBS and taking a thorough medical history and physical examination does much of the diagnosis. In fact, the most common symptom of IBS is abdominal pain and discomfort. Since these symptoms can also manifest in serious diseases like inflammatory bowel disease, it's important to know whether your symptoms are IBS or something more severe.

IBS is not a life-threatening disorder. It is very common among the general population with some estimates saying at least 1 in 5 people Americans suffer from the disorder. However, it can be physically disabling and socially embarrassing. People who have very severe IBS find it difficult to travel long distances, work a regular job, or even attend social events. On the bright side, it is not a disease and for that reason it is labelled a syndrome.

If we take a look at a normal colon, which is between the small intestine and the rectum, it receives liquid and waste from the small intestine as it makes its way out of the body. As this passes through the colon, it absorbs water and nutrients, and expels the rest out of the body as stool. Contractions in the colon are what move the faecal matter out and when this particular mechanism of the contraction of the colon muscles is irritated one can experience pain, cramping, constipation and a feeling that one has not voided properly.

CHAPTER 2

HOW DO I KNOW IF I HAVE IBS?

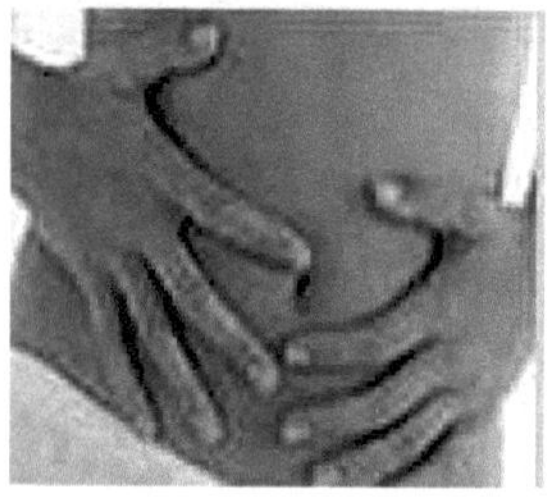

Since there is no specific medical test for IBS, you will most likely know if you have IBS by the process of elimination. There are many people with mild IBS who never go to see a physician, but if your symptoms are interfering in your ability to function or enjoy life, then you should think about visiting your physician's office to see if what you have is IBS or something that could require medical supervision.

CONVENTIONAL DIAGNOSIS

Your doctor should begin with a medical history that might pinpoint a similar issue, but with IBS, it's likely they won't notice anything with your past medical history. Your doctor will begin by eliminating some of the more serious diseases associated with the symptoms you have. These can include:

- Colon cancer
- Ovarian cancer
- Anaemia
- Inflammatory bowel disease
- An obstruction of the bowel
- Diverticulosis
- Bacterial infections
- Gallstones

To eliminate these possibilities, they will run a series of medical tests. They will request blood tests, a sedimentation rate test, and an overview of your body's chemistry profile. These will tell your doctor right away whether you are having a serious problem like kidney failure. However, it won't give them an idea as to whether you have an obstruction, colon cancer, or diverticulosis. For that reason, your doctor may request that you undergo a colonoscopy or a flexible sigmoidoscopy to get a better look at the colon and the rectum.

- **A colonoscopy** is a procedure where a long narrow tube with a light attached is used to look at the entire colon and rectum with a microscope and camera. This procedure allows your physician to take a sample of tissue for later testing. This procedure helps to pinpoint not only cancer, but abnormal growths and ulcers too.

- **A flexible sigmoidoscopy** does not include the microscope and camera and is only used to view the lower colon and rectum, as opposed to the entire colon. Many physicians believe that everyone should have their colon examined for signs of colorectal cancer yearly after they reach the age of 50. However, like any blanket recommendation, there is debate over whether this is necessary or not.

The two procedures are considered invasive and there are risks involved in having them done. You can have your colon accidentally punctured; get an infection, or experience bleeding or blood clots. If you believe you have IBS, you may need to ask your doctor whether these tests are really necessary.

Some physicians make the recommendation only when they see symptoms that are alarming, like chronic constipation or severe and persistent diarrhoea. Most IBS sufferers have sporadic episodes of constipation and diarrhoea that appear to have no rhyme or reason to them. Another reason they might order this test is if your family has a history of cancer. Only after all these other diseases are eliminated might your doctor assume you have IBS due to the process of elimination.

OTHER ALTERNATIVES FOR DIAGNOSIS

Other physicians may try to diagnose the disorder by doing some non-invasive tests first instead of going straight for the colonoscopy. The SIBO

(Small Intestine Bacterial Overgrowth) breath test was developed by Dr. Mark Pimental of the Cedars-Sinai Medical Center in Los Angeles in an effort to find out if IBS could be due to an overgrowth of bacteria in the small intestine. This is a far less invasive test than the colonoscopy or flexible sigmoidoscopy and follow-up reviews appear positive for it. In addition, there are a number of food allergy tests that can be performed to rule out possible food irritants from the diet.

SIBO TEST

This relatively new line of investigation into the potential triggers of IBS is still not widely accepted. However, the first findings in the 2004 issue of the *Journal of the American Medical Association* indicate that of IBS sufferers who experience bloating about 84% of them had abnormal readings with this test. After being treated for small intestine bacterial overgrowth, approximately 75% of them showed improvement. If you are wary of the colonoscopy or the flexible sigmoidoscopy, there are other tests available that can help with the diagnosis without being invasive. If your doctor is not aware of them, then research them on the Internet and bring that information in with you next time. Your doctor can order many of these tests directly from the manufacturing company.

FOOD INTOLERANCE TESTS

Another test that is useful for diagnosing IBS is the ELISA food test. The test is a blood test that is analyzed for sensitivity to various different foods, up to 190 different food allergies. It also has the benefit of measuring the IgG and IgE antibodies too. Unfortunately, you have to eat the food you suspect at least three days prior to taking the test otherwise the test might not be accurate. You can perform this test at home by pricking your finger and obtaining your blood sample that way. Then, send it off to a lab to have it analyzed.

At the point where they might suspect a food problem, the doctors might zero in on Celiac disease (an inability to digest wheat-based products), or anything from lactose-intolerance onwards. There are tests available to rule out other conditions like Celiac disease. Your doctor may also require that you have more antibody or food allergy tests done just to rule out those possibilities.

QUESTIONS FOR YOUR DOCTOR

So, if you show up and present yourself to your doctor and they eventually suggest that you have IBS, what questions should you ask now? First, be certain that the diagnosis is correct.
Here are some possible questions:

- Have the tests ruled out all the other possibilities?
- Does my medical history predispose me to any serious illnesses that could be the cause?
- Do you have any literature on the latest news on IBS?
- Are there any IBS support groups around?
- What do you recommend for my diet changes?
- Were there food/allergy tests done?
- Was a SIBO test performed?
- Should I schedule a follow-up after implementing dietary changes?
- Do I need medication?
- What are the potential side effects?
- Do you know of other alternatives?

All of these questions are important for ascertaining how well your doctor has investigated your problem and what your role is in now in establishing a healthier lifestyle that brings more comfort and enjoyment back to your life.

CHAPTER 3

WHAT IS THE PATHOPHYSIOLOGY OF IBS?

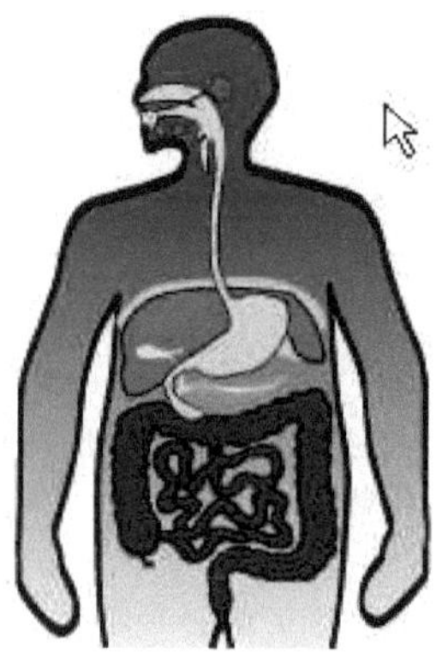

Even with a final diagnosis of an allergy or a food intolerance, it doesn't mean that you can't have both this and IBS. In fact, since the causes of IBS are unknown at this time, the signs and symptoms of IBS can be aggravated more by multiple conditions than one particular stressor. It may require that you change your lifestyle and investigate various different things for you to reclaim your health. Even if this seems a bit overwhelming, there is new information coming in daily from studies being done on IBS.

We don't know what specifically causes IBS but there is information on some correlations between particular conditions or drug usage and IBS. This can give you an idea of what might have triggered the onset at a particular time in your life. We also know that there are things that aggravate the condition that can be avoided to create more comfort.

IMMUNE SYSTEM IRRITATION

There is an enormous body of research being done to determine whether IBS might be a disorder of the immune system, instead of the digestive system. While trying to determine whether a breakdown in the immune system was responsible for IBS, there were a number of studies done to determine what the mechanism might be. Researchers began to study people who had fallen ill and been put on antibiotics to cure a particular illness. The results did not exactly point to an immune system irritation, but rather to the antibiotic use themselves.

There is some convincing evidence both in the U.S. and abroad that suggest a link between the use of antibiotics and irregular bowel symptoms. In 1998, the *European Journal of Gastroenterology and Hepatology* published a study by Mendal and Kumar, which studied 421 patients who were involved in a general health screening for IBS. It was noted that many of these patients had taken a course of antibiotics and displayed symptoms of IBS following that course of antibiotics.

A later study in 2002 in the American Journal of Gastroenterology monitored a group of patients on antibiotics for four months. This was compared to a control group that did not take any antibiotics. None of these patients had any gastrointestinal symptoms prior to visiting their doctors, however, after the course of antibiotics about 48% of the patients did display one or more symptoms of gastrointestinal upset. Only 22% of the control group displayed any such symptoms.

Also, 24% of those patients on antibiotics displayed two or more symptoms of bowel disorders, which compared to the control group rate of 6%. The final conclusion from this study what that people on antibiotics are three times more likely to report intestinal upset after a course of antibiotics, even four months after taking them.

There is ample evidence now pointing to the use of antibiotics as being a potential trigger for IBS. However, it doesn't explain why there is a correlation between IBS and antibiotics. Are the antibiotics themselves causing the disease or are the antibiotics merely affecting some part of the immune system, which then goes on to cause IBS? The jury may still be out, but more and more evidence is coming to the forefront as researchers try to find the link between antibiotic use and IBS.

WHY ANTIBIOTICS CAN TRIGGER IBS

In 2005 there was a little bit of hope for this mystery in an article published in the Journal of Clinical Gastroenterology. It stated that the use of probiotics for

IBS sufferers appeared to reduce the occurrence of symptoms in patients. This study is important because it lends credibility to the hypothesis that the reason antibiotics might trigger IBS is because they cause an imbalance in the good bacteria/bad bacteria ratios that live in the intestine.

It is estimated that over 400 species of bacteria live in the large intestine. They provide a number of valuable services. They can help to digest the food and extract nutrients. However, bacteria that cause disease can also live in the large intestine and can release toxic chemicals into your system.

It is basically a numbers game as to whether the good bacteria outnumber the bad bacteria. The good bacteria play a vital role in controlling the number of bad bacteria in the intestine. Probiotics are live cultures of bacteria beneficial to the large intestine like what is available in active yogurt cultures. By including them as dietary supplements and seeing an improvement in IBS symptoms, this hints at the potential that the good bacteria versus bad bacteria hypothesis may be correct in some cases.

ILLNESS AND IMMUNE SYSTEM DEPRESSION

It has been recognized that there does appear to be a link also for people who suffer a viral illness, food poisoning, or enteritis in the appearance of IBS symptoms. It has been theorized that the illness itself depresses the immune system, which contributes to the onset of IBS symptoms. It is also well known that the epithelium, a lining of the colon, is very much affected by the immune system as well as the nervous system. It can be highly sensitive to a number of different conditions from illness to food sensitivities and even stress. The degree of sensitivity might vary from person to person and it has been surmised that genetic factors may also play a role into why some people develop chronic IBS while others do not. It's not clear exactly how the immune system is affected, but it has been noted that the occurrence of IBS after a viral illness can be limited from between three to six months, unlike IBS affected by other causes.

FOOD SENSITIVITIES AND ALLERGIES

As mentioned earlier, there is a link between food sensitivities and allergies to the immune system hyper-response, which can lead to the appearance of IBS. The foods themselves may not cause the condition, but they do contribute greatly to the onset of symptoms. Much of this type of investigation into IBS is anecdotal and difficult to assess since most people have a variety of food sensitivities.

There is some evidence that people who suffer with Celiac disease, sensitivity to gluten or wheat-based products, can suffer with symptoms similar to IBS. In the past, before Celiac disease was recognized for what it was, many celiac patients may have been misdiagnosed with IBS instead of Celiac disease.

That is why this is one disease that needs to be eliminated when assessing a diagnosis of IBS. There is also a problem in the degree of sensitivity that people can display as well. Just because one has Celiac disease does not mean the degree of sensitivity is the same throughout the population of celiac sufferers. Some can have extreme sensitivities while others suffer only minor symptoms.

If you do suspect that a food allergy is the potential trigger for your IBS, then you will want to try to have the ELISA food test performed to identify your food triggers. This test looks for antibodies that are present when an allergic reaction is experienced with a particular food. You do have to eat the offending food three days prior to the test, however, to get accurate results.

The most common foods that people have sensitivities to are; wheat, milk, peanuts, lamb, rice, eggs, potato, soybean, tomato, pork, beef, chicken, codfish, and yeast. Of these common food allergies, it has been noticed in some studies that IBS sufferers seem to group around sensitivity to the following foods: wheat, beef, pork, lamb, and soybean. For that reason, people with IBS might be advised to eliminate beef, dairy, and wheat from their diets.

There are other foods that people might not have sensitivities or allergies to which also can affect the flora of the intestinal tract. While not showing any signs of allergic reaction to alcohol, sugar, or fats there is still evidence that these foods can either kill beneficial bacteria or change the intestinal environment to cultivate more bad bacteria. That is why even when you don't have a food allergy, a dietary approach is often recommended for sufferers of IBS. It can be as simple a change as adding more fibre to the diet to a very extreme situation like Coeliac disease where all gluten products must be avoided.

BACTERIAL OVERGROWTH

Bacterial overgrowth is blamed in situations where the bacteria may be out of control and wreaking havoc on your digestive system. Unlike the other triggers of IBS, this is one diagnosis that could be referred to as an actual cause of IBS. There is still debate over the study performed which linked bacterial overgrowth with IBS, and so the link is still tentative even though it is encouraging.

There are studies, which suggest that 92% of IBS sufferers experience bloating as a symptom after they eat. Gas is normally present when food is fermented in the intestinal tract by bacteria. If there is an overgrowth of bacteria, it could lead to excessive gas production. Using this as their basis, Dr. Lin and Dr. Pimental of Cedars-Sinai Medical Center tested a group of IBS patients with the SIBO test and found 84% of them had abnormal breath tests.

The theory here is that the overgrowth of bacteria doesn't just produce gas, but it also allows the bacteria to cross the lining of the small intestine, which is typically protected by a mucosal layer. When the bacteria proliferate to the extent that they are beginning to cross the threshold of the intestine, then the immune system is trigger. Subsequent inflammation, pain, and flu-like IBS symptoms are the result.

Ironically, the conventional treatment for IBS is a round of antibiotic treatment like rifaximin. Natural treatments consist of adding probiotic supplements to the diet or implementing a low-carbohydrate diet. There are even herbal remedies, which consist of peppermint oil, which some practitioners believe to kill bad bacteria.

If you or your doctor suspects' bacterial overgrowth, it is certainly worth taking the SIBO test as it is a far less invasive technique than a colonoscopy. Besides, colonoscopy won't detect bacterial overgrowth and is mostly for cancer and functional ailments.

STRESS

No one can escape the modern day ubiquitous presence of stress in everyday life. But, what does that have to do with IBS? Plenty, according to many studies that link too much stress to a depressed immune system. Add to that the fact that the colon is lined with nerves that are the autonomic nervous system partially controls, and you see why a spastic colon can occur with emotional or mental upset.

Normally, the nerves are there to help control the contractions as you digest and eliminate your food. When they don't work right because of extreme stress, you can experience cramps, pain, or even the sensation known as "butterflies" in the stomach.

It's important to take into account your mental and emotional health when you are looking for IBS solutions. That's why psychotherapy and massage are sometimes recommended for people with IBS. Even meditation can be helpful to alleviate the mental run-arounds that could be exhibiting themselves in a spastic colon.

While what works for one person in relieving stress may not work for another, there are a number of different options available that you can investigate. Some people like to exercise vigorously and thus relieve stress. Others prefer more relaxing forms of exercise like yoga or swimming.

If you aren't getting enough sleep, try to change your schedule to alleviate that situation. Anything that you can do to alleviate the cause of the stress in your life can help to reduce the symptoms of IBS, if stress is the major contributor. At the very least, you may come out of your battle with IBS in a more peaceful and relaxed frame of mind by seeking out different stress-relief methodologies.

HORMONES

While it seems odd to blame hormones on IBS, the sad fact is that IBS occurs twice as often in women than it does in men. This indicates some gender differences that might be linked to hormones. It is important to note that women also experience more symptoms right before their periods and after they ovulate.

The part of the cycle immediately after ovulation is associated with elevated progesterone. This can cause constipation. At the point where the post-ovulatory stage is done and the premenstrual stage begins, the progesterone suddenly declines. This is when women can experience diarrhoea.

Some studies have linked luteinizing hormone to IBS symptoms. It's also been noted that hormone replacement therapy can increase the risk of developing IBS. While menstruation can also affect IBS in predetermined manners, pregnancy and menopause aren't that clear-cut.

There is still quite a bit of investigation that needs to occur for us to understand the role of hormones in IBS development. There does appear to be a correlation between the two, but there is no evidence to suggest that the hormones themselves cause IBS.

CHAPTER 4

THE DEMOGRAPHICS OF IBS

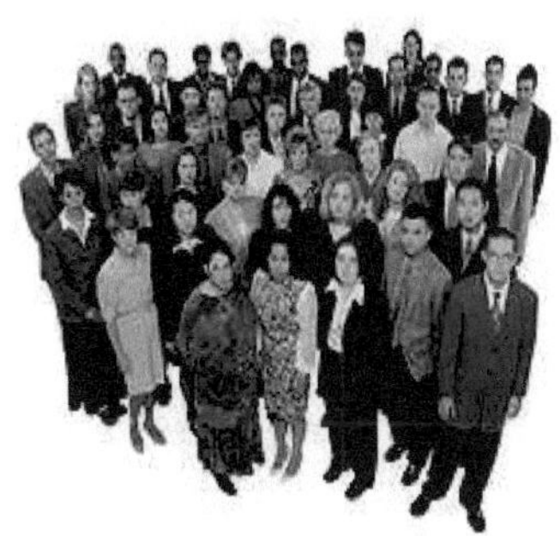

IBS is not an equal opportunity syndrome. It does target specific portions of the population. It has specific gender lines and age groupings. It even has some cultural differences. It is a very common problem, with some estimates suggesting that 1 in 5 Americans exhibiting symptoms of IBS. Worldwide, this ratio can differ. Differences in who gets IBS may depend on social and economic factors, which are difficult to measure in studies.

For instance, it is surmise that more women than men are diagnosed with IBS in the U.S. because of the social expectation that men not complain about trivial stomach complaints and to tough it out. That expectation is not the same in Asia where many more men are diagnosed with IBS than in the United States.

Economic conditions can play a factor in the syndrome by increasing stress or forcing poor dietary habits on the population. Another way the economic situation of a family can impact their willingness to be treated is that they may not have the money to seek medical attention. Thus, the problem can be under reported as well. Despite all these difficulties with the studies being done on the demographics of IBS, we have obtained a reasonable picture of the segment of the population most at risk for IBS.

WHO GETS IBS IN THE GENERAL POPULATION?

IBS generally appears in the teen years and early adulthood. It can be chronic up until Middle Ages when it begins to decline. After 50 years of age, the incidence of IBS is smaller. This doesn't mean that people who aren't between the ages of 13 to 50 will not get IBS. It actually can appear at any age, but the general population tends to congregate in the late teens to middle age years. More women than men are diagnosed with IBS in America. Some estimates suggest that 75% of all IBS sufferers are women in the United States. The same trend is not present in Asian countries, which leads many to believe that women do not actually have IBS more than men, just that men will not present themselves to a physician for treatment as often as women. However, there does appear to be a connection between hormones and IBS that might lead women to seek treatment more then men, if they experience more severe symptoms.

Worldwide, the demographics can change. While one might be tempted to suggest that the Western diet contributes to IBS, the rates of IBS are actually higher in some rural provinces of Africa than in the cities of Africa. Nigeria has the highest rate of IBS sufferers, which stood at 30% in 1997. Asian countries weren't far behind, with Japan reaching 25% prevalence of IBS in the general population and China with 23%.

There may be some validity to the idea that genetics can play a role in the development of IBS. It is known that many African Americans have an enzyme deficiency that makes them lactose intolerant. This can produce symptoms similar to IBS. Native Americans also have this genetic characteristic. People who suffer with Coeliac disease, an inability to digest gluten, also have a genetic predisposition to that sensitivity.

It appears some people's colons are just more sensitive than other people's colons. While this isn't much help to you if you are African-American, it can help you to pinpoint what your problem might be if you belong to a particular ethnic group that has genetic tendencies that don't allow the digestion of certain foods. Then, you can simply choose to eliminate that food from your diet or substitute it with a different food.

WHAT ABOUT CHILDREN? (PEDIATRIC IBS)

There are instances of childhood IBS even if the physician may not want to diagnose it as such. Instead, it might be diagnosed as encopresis, which is really another form of IBS in children. The symptoms of encopresis are similar to IBS in that you might have involuntary soiling or chronic constipation after a child is toilet-trained. It is estimated that 1 to 2% of children under 10 years of age are diagnosed with encopresis.

While the conventional physician may not see a connection between IBS and encopresis, it might be caused by some of the same problems: food allergies or a round of antibiotic treatments. What is usually prescribed for children who have bowel movement problems are laxatives, enemas, or both. A schedule of potty sitting times is also recommended to try to help stabilize the child's bowel movements.

In cases where no functional problem can be determined, it is sometimes suggested that the child might be exhibiting a psychological disorder that is characterized by defiance or oppositional behaviour.

In the very young, the idea that a baby is trying to be defiant would seem a little odd. Yet, some of the same symptoms that young children exhibit and are labelled encopresis for young children are also displayed in young infants. Colicky babies may be experiencing a form of IBS, which can be exacerbated by food allergies too.

Certain foods are contraindicated for all babies due to potential severe reactions. These are: nuts, eggs, milk, soy, fish, citrus fruits, food additives, and shellfish (shrimp and other crustaceans). If there are other foods that appear to be causing your baby distress, you can have it tested by a paediatric allergist to verify your suspicions.

<u>*CHAPTER 5*</u>

OTHER TREATMENTS FOR IBS

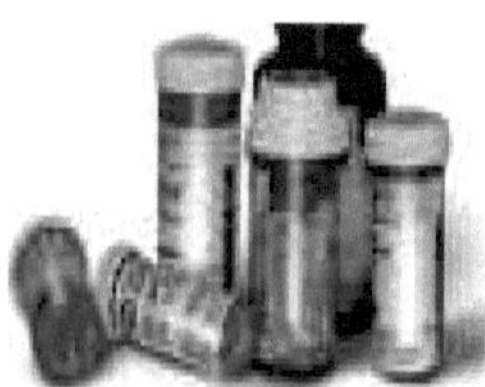

In book 2 of this series entitled "**IBS and Nutrition, *The Nutritional Approach To Managing Irritable Bowel Syndrome (IBS)*"**, I go into great detail about various diets and how they are used to treat IBS. So, we won't go into great discussion about it here. It would be a good idea to purchase a copy since it is a key part of the overall treatment plan for controlling IBS.

However, diet is not the only way to treat IBS, even if it is the most common approach. IBS is said to affect the nervous system, the intestines, and the immune system. For that, there has to be more than one approach. There is a wide range of treatment options available that you can explore as you begin to establish a diet program. These should complement your dietary approach and not replace it completely.

- **Conventional medications** can rely on laxatives for constipation or enemas for diarrhea. Also, there are a number of antibiotics being used with IBS. Antispasmodics are also used to keep the colon from being spastic. Some people are even put on antidepressants to help resolve some of the issues with IBS.

- **Natural supplements** can run the gamut from psyllium within natural fiber supplements to herbs and vitamins. Popular herbs to treat IBS are peppermint, chamomile, and fennel. These all can be taken in different forms whether tea or supplements.

- **Probiotics** are an entire natural field onto themselves. There are companies whose sole mission is to sell probiotic supplements and food products. However, probiotics are available naturally in many foods without having to pay higher prices for special brands.

- **Alternative therapies** have also been explored with the addition of acupuncture and hypnotherapy to help with IBS symptoms. We will briefly discuss these two options as well.

- **Stress relief** – Psychotherapy is the conventional means of dealing with an emotional or mental trauma. However, you don't have to shell out tons of money for a good psychotherapist to get some stress relief. You can learn to meditate or instead opt for a massage.

- **Exercise** - Something that is rarely discussed with regards to IBS is exercise. Any health program can be aided with the addition of exercise and IBS is no different. Instead of strenuous, stressful exercise programs though you might want to take up more relaxing and soothing activities. You can learn how to do yoga (which will help in your meditation practice) or you can even learn Tai Chi. Don't limit yourself to a standard aerobics class, especially if you don't think you can get through the class without having to take a break in the middle.

CONVENTIONAL MEDICATIONS

If you have tried adding more fiber to your diet and your IBS is not responding to it, then you might want to see what other options you have to relieve your symptoms. Conventional medications treat constipation with laxatives and diarrhea with medications to stop diarrhea or antispasmodics (muscle relaxers). The problem with IBS is that it often alternates between bouts of diarrhea and bouts of constipation. Unless you have more episodes of one than another, it may be difficult for your doctor to give you one medication that doesn't affect the other symptoms adversely.

If these fail to show any improvement, a conventional doctor might try an antibiotic or an antidepressant too. The idea is to target a bacterial infection or maybe even that your symptoms are more about an emotional or mental upset. Remember that conventional medicine doesn't really know or acknowledge the causes of IBS. Though there is ample evidence to suggest that an overgrowth of bacteria could cause the problem, it is not a foregone conclusion in the medical world. There need to be more tests done before this information becomes more widely accepted. Until then, the doctors will stick with their conventional approaches, which are bound to be trial and error since no cause has been determined. Instead, they will try to treat the symptoms and hope one of the medicines they prescribes works. However, they will most likely start with the easier solutions first, even when treating only symptoms

LAXATIVES AND ANTI-DIARRHEALS

That's why natural laxatives are always prescribed first. They are gentler on your system and work to bulk up the stool too. This makes them helpful for diarrhea as well. We already discussed natural laxatives like Metamucil that contains psyllium and others like Acacia fibers. An overuse of over-the-counter laxative products has been shown to create more problems. They aren't meant to be used long-term and can create additional problems with chronic constipation or a dysfunctional colon being the final result.

Other conventional medications are known by their brand names. These are:

- **Loperamide** – A drug used for the treatment of diarrhea.
- **Mebeverine** – A drug that is used to calm the colon and considered an antispasmodic.
- **Imodium** – Used to treat diarrhea and is available over-the-counter.
- **Milk of Magnesia** – Also used to treat diarrhea and is also available over-the-counter. It is the gentlest of all the over-the-counter laxatives, however, it is also not recommended for long-term use.
- **Senokot** – A laxative, over-the-counter drug.

- **ExLax –** A laxative, over-the-counter drug.
- **Lotronex –** Prescribed for diarrhea-predominant IBS.
- **Zelnorm –** Prescribed for constipation-predominant IBS.
- **Codeine –** Prescribed for mild diarrhea-predominant IBS.
- **Librax –** An anti-anxiety drug prescribed for IBS.

The way conventional medications work is to treat the symptoms instead of trying to locate the cause. However, even symptom relief can have its limits. Many of these medications can cause other side effects, if taken long-term. These are a just a few of the brand names of medications available for IBS sufferers. There are many more types of medications available from antidepressants to antibiotics as well.

ANTIDEPRESSANTS

While it may seem odd to prescribe and antidepressant for a colon disorder, the reasoning is that a spastic colon is affected by the nervous system. By reducing the stress and strain of mental and emotional turmoil in a patient, a conventional doctor hopes to calm the spastic colon into behaving. At the very least, it can help the patient to continue with the syndrome without being too upset about it.

Some of these products are prescribed for a long period of time to many patients before they are found to have some serious side effects and then withdrawn from the market. Zelnorm is one such product, which was withdrawn by the FDA due to an increase in heart problems in patients that were prescribed the drug.

As of now, there are drugs that target serotonin levels that are being prescribed for IBS. These drugs are called Selective serotonin reuptake inhibitor antidepressants or SSRIs for short. Therapists to treat anxiety and personality disorders typically use them. They can also treat clinical depression.

People taking SSRIs have a 1 to 4 week adjustment period. During that time a number of different side effects can appear, the most serious being ideations of suicide, liver failure, or renal impairment. The less serious side effects are nausea, dizziness, headaches, and a change in appetite.

There are natural antidepressants like Saint John's Wort that have been used in European countries for years for depression. There are currently some studies being undertaken to see if it can also help people who are diagnosed with IBS. One of the positive factors about natural herbal remedies is that they tend to have fewer side effects than chemical conventional medications. However, some claim this is because herbal remedies are not as well documented as conventional medications.

ANTIBIOTICS

Recently, it has been theorized that antibiotics might be helpful for an overgrowth of bacteria in the gut. Studies indicate that Rifaximin might be a good treatment for IBS that is characterized by bloating and flatulence. One thing that doesn't seem to be addressed is how an antibiotic can be a cure for IBS when there is also evidence suggesting that IBS appears more often in people who have just undergone a course in antibiotics. It is possible that one antibiotic causes the overgrowth by killing off good bacteria and another might make the environment more favorable thus re-establishing a balance. However, this approach is very new and with any new treatments they are roughly experimental.

NATURAL SUPPLEMENTS

Natural supplements are very widespread and their usage tested on generations of people who had no conventional medicine at the time. Their effectiveness may be debated, and their usefulness may be an individual matter, but the folklore of natural herbs and supplements is one of the richest sources of healing on the planet. There's no reason to ignore it in favor of conventional medicines, particularly if they do happen to work for you.

Side effects with natural herbs and supplements are usually not severe, unlike conventional medications. They are gentler on your system and sometimes require you to take them for a longer period of time to get some benefit from them. The advantage in being that gentle is that there is less risk of having a severe side effect. Be aware though that just because something is natural and herbal does not mean that you can't have a reaction to it. Please read up on any herb you are considering ingesting to make sure you understand the risks. There are some herbs that are very powerful and dangerous, but still quite available to the general public.

For the most part, you don't have to worry too much with IBS. Most of the herbs, supplements, and vitamins are safe for everyone. They consist of treatments that even conventional medicines add to their over-the-counter products, like psyllium. Peppermint also is being used in capsules to help alleviate IBS symptoms. Even minerals can be used for their special properties. High doses of vitamin C can also be used as a natural laxative.

NATURAL FIBER

Well, the first line of defense whether natural or conventional is a natural product: psyllium. It is present in Metamucil and Konsyl. It works for both diarrhea and constipation. However, some people are very sensitive to psyllium and have to go with something gentler. That's where Acacia fiber comes in. This is also a natural fiber that can be added to the diet to help relieve some of the symptoms of IBS.

As discussed earlier, fiber supplements are being marketed in many forms. You no longer have to drink down a gritty drink in order to increase the fiber in your diet. There are wafer and capsule forms of fiber supplements. Just be careful that whatever product you pick it doesn't aggravate food sensitivity. Many of them have sugar in them and the wafers are full of gluten.

Another source of fiber that is available in most health food stores is whole flax seed. Flax seed is considered a wonder food for its many healthful properties. It is not only an excellent source of fiber, but it is high in Omega-3 fatty acids. This one supplement that can help you reduce your bad cholesterol. This is a very bountiful source of antioxidants, compounds that are known to reduce the signs of aging. They work to fight free radicals that cause all kinds of bodily deterioration. As if that weren't enough, flax seeds are high in manganese and shock full of B vitamins.

Flax oil is available for people who want to include the health benefits of flax seed without the fiber. However, you want to include the fiber as well as the other health benefits. For that, you will need to buy the whole seed and either dress your salads and smoothies with it or learn how to crush it in a mill so you can eat it by the spoonful in the morning.

HERBAL REMEDIES FOR IBS

By far the most common herbal remedy for IBS is peppermint. It is a natural antispasmodic and can alleviate pain too. You can take peppermint in an herbal tea or as enteric-coated capsules right before meals. The coating keeps them from dissolving in the stomach where they could cause additional stomach upset. Instead, they are created to dissolve in the intestine where their antispasmodic and pain-killing properties work to your advantage. Even the Altoids peppermint candies can help you get some of those soothing qualities when you need them the most.

Just be very careful that you aren't susceptible to peppermint sensitivity. People who have acid reflux disease shouldn't take peppermint because it can trigger that disease. If that's the case with you, you can avoid peppermint and try something like fennel, ginger, or chamomile instead.

Fennel is used to relieve bloating and gas. It can even help relieve menstrual cramps, which make it ideal for women who have worse IBS symptoms near their periods. Fennel has antibacterial properties, which may be one of the reasons it helps IBS sufferers. It is also anti-inflammatory. Fennel has a delicious licorice-like flavor and can be used in teas, entrees, and even as an after dinner mint like Indians use. They are chewed and eaten whole and can help you deal with some of the more difficult and embarrassing problems with IBS: bloating and gas. You do want to include fennel everyday in your diet, whether as a tea or in some other way.

Along with fennel, ginger is known to aide the digestion. It has been used for centuries to relieve cramps and nausea too. Ginger works very well in some ethnic cuisines like Thai. It can be bought as a crystallized candy and eaten that way. It makes a great tea, along with fennel, and anise seed.

Chamomile is basically to calm the nerves. It works as an antispasmodic and a natural sedative. Some people have sensitivities to chamomile that also have sensitivities to hay fever. So, as usual, be careful before you engage a new treatment, whether it is natural or conventional. Chamomile is most often taken internally as a tea although it has a lovely fragrance and can be used in aromatherapy to relieve insomnia.

Regardless of what herb you choose, be sure that your conventional doctor knows what you are taking. Herbs, in some cases, can interact with conventional prescriptions or even block the benefits of other prescriptions. In order for your physician to get a wide view of your treatment, do not hide the fact that you're thinking of taking herbal medications. Instead, make him or her a partner in your decision. That way, if you are also taking a conventional medication, they may be more alert to possible interactions with your herbal regimen.

PROBIOTICS

Probiotics are natural microorganisms that are live cultures in foods. They help to re-establish the colony of good bacteria in the intestine once it has been wiped out by a course of antibiotics or some other imbalance. They are evident in fermented products like yogurts and sour milk. They are used to treat diarrhea and to help boost the immune system.

It wouldn't seem that you can get a live culture in a dry product, but you actually can. This has spurred a large market for people selling probiotic cultures in capsule form. There are also liquid and tablet forms of probiotics. They are available either directly from the distributor online or in natural health food stores.

There are specialty foods now being marketed to consumers with probiotics. Kombucha tea is a Korean-type of fermented tea available at some whole foods stores that is high in probiotics. As the trends towards more functional foods increase, you will probably notice more foods touting the benefits of probiotics on their labels.

ALTERNATIVE THERAPIES

With our growing understanding that the mind affects the body and vice-versa, there are many more consumers interested in holistic approaches to their ailments. Irritable bowel syndrome is no different. Patients may decide to try alternative therapies in conjunction with conventional medicines to complement the physical approach with a more mental/emotional/spiritual connection.

Acupuncture is an alternative therapy that requires a bit of faith in energetic medicine. Acupuncturists believe that the body has an energetic system that can become blocked and result in disease. Energy lines called meridians take the energy called chi and distribute it to varying parts of the body. When chi does not flow well, then you have disease.

For that reason, they use needles to help the flow of chi enter areas associated with the digestive system. This may not be your intestine! It might be a spot on your toe or even on your face. The needles are said not to hurt too much and this ancient treatment is well respected in China. It is even used to alleviate pain quite successfully.

Hypnotherapy is used to place the patient in an altered state where they can use their mind power to resolve some of the symptoms of IBS. A skilled hypnotherapist may be required although some people use tapes that they play to help them achieve the necessary state of consciousness. In that state, suggestions are given to either relax the colon or to help alleviate symptoms associated with IBS.

Costs for acupuncture and hypnotherapy may be on the high end and they are usually not covered by medical insurance, unless you have a special alternative policy like some Blue Cross and Blue Shield programs. The duration of treatment varies from person to person, but it does require multiple visits.

Like acupuncture, hypnotherapy requires an open-mind. It has proven successful for many people, but if it's not your thing, then don't stress out. Some people are more easily hypnotized than others. Some people don't like the idea of sticking needles into their body, even when it might resolve their IBS symptoms.

If you don't like the idea of hypnotherapy or acupuncture, you don't have to try them. They are offered here to give a very well rounded view of the many different types of treatments available to IBS sufferers. There are still even more approaches available for people trying to win their battle with IBS and it's expected that as more and more research is done that these will be added to in the near future.

In our final section, we will discuss the immense area of stress relief. The connection between the body and mind are crucial for releasing some of the anguish, anxiety, and emotional upset that can occur with IBS. In addition, it has been shown to be helpful physically too.

STRESS RELIEF

If you have IBS, you have stress. There is no two ways about it. Whether the stress came first and then the IBS or whether it was the other way around, at this point, it probably doesn't matter. The stress of having a syndrome like IBS can wear on you day after day. It's important for your mental and emotional health to take time to ease some of the stress in your life before it becomes debilitating.

LIGHTEN YOUR LOAD

Although IBS is not going to lead to a disease like heart disease or cancer, you do need to treat yourself with a little more loving kindness. Attempt to modify those areas of your life that you are able to change to make them less stressful for you. This cannot only keep you from becoming ill with stress-induced diseases but also it can make you enjoy your life more.

Try to determine some of the things that bring you some peace of mind. It is different for everyone. Here are a few examples of some possible stress relief strategies for when things are becoming too much to bear:

- Count to ten
- Take a warm bath
- Do some aromatherapy
- Light some candles and lower the lights
- Listen to soft music
- Read
- Pray
- Write down some positive affirmations
- Take a short walk
- Drink some water
- Breathe deeply
- Count your blessings

- Hear a joke
- Tell a joke
- Garden
- Smell the flowers
- Hug your children

These are all small things that can be done on the spur of the moment to help you reduce stress in your life. When you start to put your issues into perspective, you may find the joy re-entering your life. Half the battle is the attitude you choose to have about your condition and the stressful conditions around you.

LEARN TO MANAGE YOUR TIME

One of the things that contribute to a stressful life is a lack of planning. The more you learn how to manage your time and plan for the potential problems, the more prepared and in control you will feel. If you do not have good organization and time management skills then this is the time to learn. You will want to learn how to write a **"to do"** list and how to keep track of events on a calendar, at the very least.

Try to keep your work area or your house area clutter-free. Simply disposing of clutter can help you feel more organized. Keep to the rule that if you are not using it, and then it can be disposed of or given away. Try to keep your environments to the bare minimums and you will have less to clean in the long run.

Part of learning how to manage your time is recognizing that you can say no. Many people become stressed out because they commit themselves to too many projects. Instead of learning to say no without shrinking or apologizing, they are left with little time for themselves because they are too busy pleasing others. If you are a people-pleaser take a look at the commitments you've made. Are they adding to your stress level? Is it essential that you be the one to do a particular task? Might someone else be better at it? Can you pay someone to do it for you?

You may balk at the idea of paying someone to do something you can do yourself. But, in time management this is a very clever strategy. You have to realize that your time is worth a set amount of money based on the skills that you have developed. If it costs you an hour to make $35, then it pays to hire someone to come and clean your home at $15/hr or less.

You still end up making money and you have less stress too. There's no reason to put yourself out trying to do too many things just because you think you are expected to do them Instead hire some help or recruit your family to help you manage the household.

Children don't often take to household chores unless you make it a habit. Make it clear that everyone dirties the house and everyone should be involved in cleaning it. Your time should be just as valuable as anyone else's time in the family. And, you should set aside time for yourself to help you de-stress and relax. However, you will never get to that stage if your life is full of clutter, you are trying to meet to many other people's demands, and you have not organized your time to make the best use of it.

Learning how to manage your time is a skill that can be learned by reading articles on time management. It's not something that takes a lot of insight or cleverness. It just takes the willingness to prioritize your time at home so that your life becomes less stressful and more manageable. This, in turn, can translate into a healthier, happier you.

FOCUS ON RELAXING DURING "ME" TIME

Okay, so you've laid down the ground rules and made it clear that you need some "me" time. Now, you might have a half hour or twenty minutes in the day to help you focus on relaxing. This can seem like a simple proposition, but actually people who have gotten into a habitual lifestyle of always hurrying find it very difficult to settle down. Take a deep breath. This is going to be a lifestyle change and eventually you will enjoy it and wonder how you ever got to the point where you were wound up tight as a spinning top.

One of the first things you can do to help to release some of the anxiety of a totally occupied mind is to learn how to meditate. Meditation is very easy to do. There are workshops that teach a variety of different meditation techniques. You probably want to stick with something that relaxes you but doesn't put you too much into an altered state of mind.

For that, reserve a quiet corner in your house. You can sit on the floor on a cushion or pillow, or you can choose to sit a chair. Keep your back straight and erect. Close your eyes and breathe deeply. Then, just try to watch your breath. Stay with your breath. When it comes in, notice it coming in. When it goes out, notice the exhalation. Try to keep your mind on your breath and this will soon lead to your mind quieting down and getting stiller.

What typically happens to people who are new to meditation and who are used to being terminally busy is that they sit down for a few minutes and then start to fidget. There mind goes speeding down the highway at the same speed it's always gone. The person has a difficult time sticking with the breath and one thought leads to another and pretty soon you've forgotten all about the breath. Don't worry, this is pretty common. Just say to yourself: "Thinking, thinking" and thus notice the thinking. Or mention what it is you are thinking to yourself like "cat" or "dog" or whatever the object of your mental fantasy is, then bring the attention softly back to the breath. By pulling your attention back to the breath you can eventually tame the mind from running away with itself.

Try to limit your meditation to twenty minutes every other day when you begin and only slowly increase it, as you are comfortable. Remember that you aren't trying to achieve anything in particular. You don't do it right if your mind settles down and you aren't doing it wrong if it doesn't. Don't make your meditation practice another competition or you will find yourself stressing out over your meditation practice. Instead, keep it light and don't worry too much about whether it's working or not. The fact is, you are sitting still for a little while and that will help you to relax and produce a slower rhythm to your life.

There are a number of different types of meditation, as mentioned before. You can try progressive relaxation, if that suits you better. In this practice the key is to slowly relax each muscle in your body consciously until the entire body is sitting still and relaxed. Progressive relaxation is easy to learn and there are books that teach the practice. You can also get audiotapes that will walk you through the process.

These types of techniques are great for people who have anxiety with their IBS. It can help them to see that the mind does not control them, they control the mind. It can also give a feeling of being in control for a short period of the day, which can spread out to make them more confident during the rest of the day.

TAKING TIME OUT FOR A MASSAGE

If you've never treated yourself to a massage, now is the time to try one! Massage isn't just about feeling good, although it does make you feel exceedingly well. There is an entire theory that surrounds massage that suggests that the muscles of the body store emotional and mental traumas in the muscles of the body. By massaging different areas of the body, those traumas can be released as toxins, which can then be flushed out by drinking plenty of water afterwards.

Like meditation, there are a number of different types of massage techniques available to choose from. If you don't like one type, that doesn't mean you can't try a different one. When you first show up, your massage therapist may ask you why you are there. You can say stress or you can indicate IBS, because this information will help him or her decide which areas to concentrate on and which to avoid.

Massage is done partially clothed in some cases. They may offer you a towel to place around your private parts before you get on the table. The room should be slightly warm and the table shouldn't be cold either. They may ask you if you prefer one type of oil to another. Lavender scented oils are great for calming the nerves, if you are so inclined.

You can opt for a ½ hour massage or a full hour massage. You probably won't want to be doing anything strenuous after your massage. Be careful driving your vehicle too as you may be pretty spaced out after you leave. Always remember to drink lots of water after a massage session to clear out the toxins that might have been released. This is not only good for the massage treatment but is helpful for your IBS too.
A typical massage can range from $60 to $100/hour. It all depends on what type of massage you are getting and whom you are getting it from. You can get some deals for massages at times, if you know someone, or they are learning the art and need guinea pigs. Massage therapists are professionals that have to be licensed in their state to practice. So, their services are not cheap, but they are worth it.

WHAT ABOUT PSYCHOTHERAPISTS?

A trained psychotherapist can help you deals with symptoms of depression that may arise because of your IBS. Psychologists are also able to prescribe antidepressants, if you think you want to go that route. You will want to get a referral and see if your insurance will cover a trip to see a psychotherapist.

You will want to get a psychotherapist that specializes in the particular symptoms you are trying to address. If you have insomnia, then seek out one that deals with sleep disorders as well as depression. Be aware that each psychotherapist is different and can come with their own allegiance to different schools of thought. If you get a referral from your physician they can give you an idea of what to expect when you visit a psychotherapist.

Talk therapy is usually what most psychotherapists engage in. This may seem a roundabout way to treat a digestive disorder, but some patients benefit from it. If you find it doesn't work for you, you might want to still take advantage of mental health services by seeing if there is a local IBS support group you can join. Sometimes a group format can be more beneficial than one-on-one sessions with a psychotherapist.

DO I HAVE TO EXERCISE?

There's no hard and fast rule that says you have to exercise to get rid of IBS. What is known is that people that include exercise in their daily routines are healthier. It doesn't require you to be an Olympic athlete to get some of the benefits of exercising. You can include 20 minutes of aerobic exercise like walking and still find yourself feeling better.

Exercise can also affect your eating habits. If you are busy swimming, you have less time for snacking. Also, people who exercise seem to suffer less from depression. Exercise is said to be a mood enhancer and is believed to help release chemicals in the brain that make people happier.

Another benefit of exercise for IBS patients is that any exercise, even gentle ones like yoga, can get the bowel to return to a normal pattern of contractions. It works the muscles of bowel when you are exercising and this can strengthened your digestive system.

If you are looking for a specific exercise to work the colon and to give some relief from spasms, then try bent-knee sit-ups. You can get a simple exercise mat and start your IBS exercise program today. It doesn't take joining a gym or becoming a marathon runner. Just include some daily exercise into your routine and start seeing the difference as you continue with the program. The worse that can happen is that you'll gain some muscle and lose some fat.

YOGA FOR IBS

If you want something that kills two birds with one stone for IBS, it's yoga. Yoga is a meditative exercise that can both strengthen your muscles and help aide in meditation practice. Yoga is a taught as a series of postures that increase flexibility and stamina. You don't start off knowing how to contort your body into pretzel shapes, but eventually you build up that endurance.

If you were never someone who liked aerobic classes or working out with weights, then yoga might be the ticket for you. The focus is still on the breath in yoga. You are preparing yourself for the meditation by beginning to take up the appropriate postures. Some of these postures are simple stretches and others are more complex.

You could probably learn yoga using an instructional video. There is a number of great yoga teachers that can help you master some of the poses and can offer some helpful suggestions while you practice in their class. You can't get that from a video. It is better to join a class and learn how to do the poses correctly rather than practice the poses incorrectly and possibly risk hurting yourself.

TAI CHI

Tai Chi is a graceful set of flowing movements that help to build stamina and endurance. They also have a meditative-like quality and can relieve stress. People in China can be seen practicing this ancient martial art in large groups. Unfortunately, in the U.S. and other countries it may be harder to find an instructor.

If you do have an interest in learning Tai Chi, you might be able to pick it up from instructional material. It does work with the breath as well as movement and the subtleties of the practice may be lost though. It is probably better to find an instructor if you can. Even though it is difficult to find them in some areas of the country, this is one practice that is legendary for its health benefits.

Tai Chi is a useful stress management exercise, which is supposed to increase a person's vitality and health. Even if you are not interested in this type of martial art, you will be fascinated by the flowing moving meditation. It is beautiful to watch and makes you want to join in.

PUTTING THINGS INTO PERSPECTIVE

Having irritable bowel syndrome is not a welcome diagnosis. On the one hand it means a chronic condition that can be difficult to treat. The causes are still a bit of a mystery and the treatments vary widely. On the other hand, once you have a diagnosis of IBS, you know what you are dealing with. You don't have a degenerative disease and there is hope that you can recover and get better.

There may not be one single pill that your doctor can prescribe that will get rid of all your symptoms. It may be a bit frustrating as you work out a new lifestyle that helps you control the IBS. The benefits though are multiple. By choosing to take control of your health and diet, you will not only be alleviating your IBS symptoms but you could also affect your health in the long-term. Many of the diets and behaviors outlined in this e-book can impact your risk of getting cancer, diabetes, and heart disease too.

So, being forced to start early in managing your health can be a mixed blessing. It's not fun to have IBS. It can be embarrassing and inconvenient. It can make you depressed. It can affect your lifestyle and make it difficult to schedule anything. The good news is that this may all be temporary. Once you get a handle on the triggers that are causing the appearance of IBS in your life, you will be able to remove them and substitute healthier behaviors.

This can lead to improvements in overall health, fitness, and mental and emotional well-being. You may find that your IBS was a wake-up call that put your life back in order after all was said and done. You can be happy knowing that the syndrome that made you uncomfortable could be the reason you've extended your lifespan, avoided other major diseases, and found all natural treatments that put you back in control of your own life.

Part 2 ""**IBS and Nutrition, *The Nutritional Approach To Managing Irritable Bowel Syndrome (IBS)"***. It is a key part of the overall plan to control IBS

IBS and Nutrition

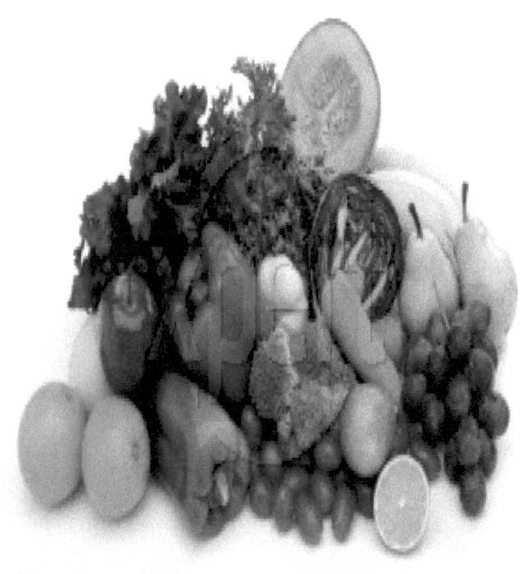

The Nutritional Approach To Managing Irritable Bowel Syndrome (IBS)

Belinda Asonganyi

CHAPTER 6

NUTRITIONAL APPROACH TO IBS

THE IMPORTANCE OF NUTRITION IN CONTROLLING IBS

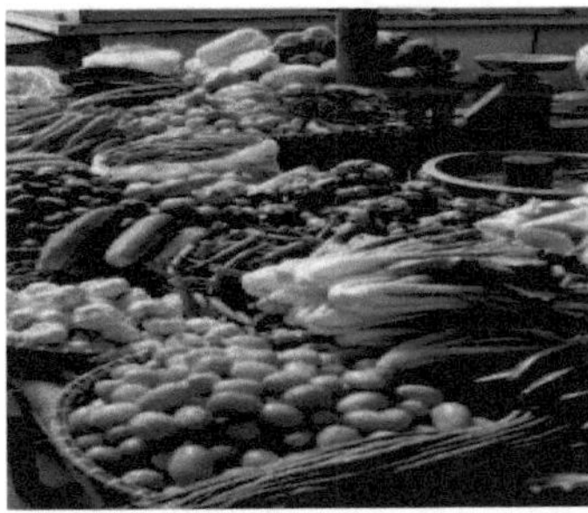

ISB (irritable Bowel Syndrome) affects approximately 45-million Americans and up to 12% of those over age 50. It is more common than heart disease, diabetes, depression, or asthma. For some people with IBS, symptoms are no more than an annoying but manageable nuisance.

The good news is that IBS can be managed effectively through a change in diet. Good nutrition is a key element in managing IBS. However, it is not the only element used to manage IBS. Used in combination with the appropriate medications, counselling and stress reduction techniques, the nutritional approach (change in dietary habits) will make the difference between controlling your IBS and struggling to gain control of it.

Ways to manage IBS nutritionally are:

- To eat a varied diet that includes high-fibre foods
- Drink plenty of water
- Avoid foods that make you feel worse

DIETARY CHANGES FOR IBS

If you have mild to moderate IBS, it is necessary to make some changes to your diet in an effort to control your IBS. Many people find that their IBS symptoms become worse after they eat. Sometimes certain foods make symptoms worse.

However, no particular foods cause everyone with IBS to have symptoms. Doctors do not advocate a particular diet to manage symptoms. Instead it comes down to trial and error where many people find that they feel better when they stop eating certain foods. These foods may cause the intestines to contract, which can aggravate IBS in people who have diarrhoea as their main symptom.

NOTE: Those who suffer with severe **IBS** may need additional help in the form of medication etc.

This book will help to find alternative foods to replace the ones that you had to give up. It also has some great recipes for foods that do not trigger IBS episodes. You can try any or all of them and I am sure that if you do, you will love them. Best of all, I bet you won't feel cheated out of not being able to eat certain foods, but rather you will feel just as satisfied. Also try experimenting with foods you can have from the list in the section of this book that defines foods that will not trigger IBS. You can get as creative as you want when planning your meals or creating new recipes to enjoy. By combining foods that you can have from our list, you will have a variety of new dishes to try. Go ahead and enjoy!

As I just said earlier, you may not know what is triggering an episode until you eat something and have it set off your IBS. That is why it is so important to keep a food diary or journal to keep track of what you are eating and what type of reaction if any you have after you eat it.

To help you keep track of the foods you eat, I have included a "Food Journal" sheet at the end of this book that you can print out and use to record the foods you eat and the reaction you may or may not have gotten. Keeping a diary of food intake and symptoms can assist in identifying foods that trigger your symptoms.

Use the journal daily and once a week; review it to see when you had an episode and what foods you were eating at the time. This will help you to rid your diet of these foods and have fewer episodes or maybe even get rid of the problem for good. Another good reason for the diary is that it can be reviewed with your doctor to identify problem areas and possible treatment options.

CHAPTER 7

DIET PLANS

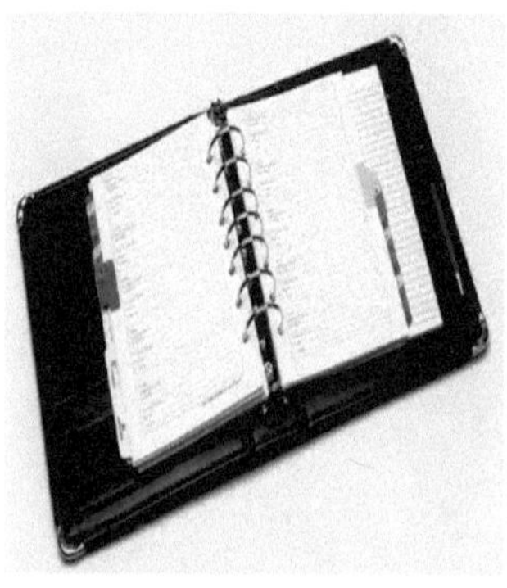

THE RIGHT FOODS TO EAT

There are many types of foods available the will not trigger and IBS episode. In this section, I will share them with you so that you may try some or all of them to see what works for you. I do need to ***caution*** you here that you should always speak with a medical professional before making any type of changes to your diet.

A drastic change in your eating habits may do you more harm than good. Try introducing one new food item at a time and record the reaction. If you have a reaction from the food, stop eating it and move to the next choice and so on until you find a balance of foods that can be eaten without causing IBS to trigger. Try eating more protein-rich foods as well.

This is where your food journal sheet located at the end of this book will come in handy. Print a copy or several copies and begin journaling what you eat and what the reaction was. It is important to introduce only a few of these types of foods at once. Don't try to change too much too soon; it can actually work against you.

Just remember that different people can have different triggers for their IBS symptoms. You may try eliminating foods or beverages one at a time to see whether symptoms improve. If a specific food does not seem to be related to symptoms, there is no need to continue avoiding it.

Fibre in your diet

Before we get to the right foods to eat list, let's talk about fibre in your diet. You can find fibre in fruits, vegetables, whole-grain breads, and cereals. It is a good idea to introduce some fibre into your daily diet plan because:

1. It improves the way the intestines work
2. It may also reduce bloating, pain, and other symptoms

A word of caution is necessary here. Make sure that you introduce fiber into you diet very slowly! Too much fiber introduced too soon can cause a myriad of problems that include bloating and excessive gas, so a little at a time is the best way to go.

problems associated with IBS.

There are 2 types of fibre: ***soluble and insoluble***. Soluble fibre is in the form of fruits, vegetables and supplements. **Soluble** fibre helps both diarrhoea and constipation. It dissolves in water and forms a gel-like material. Soluble fibre is the key to preventing the abdominal spasms and bowel dysfunction of IBS. This is true not just for soluble fibre foods but supplements as well. Clinical studies with IBS patients have repeatedly proven the benefits of soluble fibre and soluble fibre supplements. Soluble fibre will, in fact, work beautifully to keep your GI tract running smoothly, comfortably and pain-free on a day-to-day basis.

Insoluble fibre is in the form of many foods (see foods high in fibre list further down in this section). It helps constipation by moving material through your digestive system and adding bulk to your stool. It will help eliminate painful diarrhoea episodes by adding substance to stools.

Soluble fibre food sources

Soluble fibre is found in foods such as:

- Dried beans and other legumes
- Oats
- Barley
- Berries

Foods are high in fibre

Here are some good sources of fibre filled foods. Eating foods from any of these groups will help add fibre to your diet.

- Fruits
- Vegetables
- Whole grain bread
- Whole grain cereals
- Barley
- Black beans
- Bran cereal
- Brown rice
- Dry fruits
- Flaxseed meal
- Fresh fruit with skins (may be better tolerated cooked or canned)
- Fresh vegetables (may be better tolerated cooked)
- Garbanzo beans
- Kidney beans
- Lentils
- Lima beans
- Navy beans
- Nuts
- Oats
- Raisins
- Soybeans
- Split peas
- Whole grains, including breads and cereals
- Yams
- Probiotics, like the healthy bacteria found in yogurt or in probiotic supplements, may help decrease symptoms of IBS. Adding yogurt to your diet may help ease symptoms of irritable bowel syndrome (IBS), according to some research.
- Try a lactose-free diet to see if bloating and gas decrease
- Eating a low-fat diet will also help with the symptoms of IBS

Other sources of fibre

In addition to eating fibre-rich food, you can increase fibre intake by taking bulk-forming supplements such as:

- Methylcellulose (Citrucel)
- Polycarbophil (Equalactin, FiberCon, Mitrolan)
- Psyllium (Fiberall, Konsyl-D, Metamucil)

Remember that as you increase fibre in your diet, it is also important to drink more liquids (water and decaffeinated beverages). Aim for 6 to 8 glasses of water per day. Keep your body as hydrated as possible to make the fibre work better within your body. Too little fluids can be an issue when adding fibre to your diet, so remember to drink fluids often.

Soluble Fibre Supplements

The most common soluble fibre supplements are:

- Acacia Tummy Fibre
- Equalactin,
- FiberChoice
- Fibersure
- Benefiber
- Metamucil
- Konsyl
- Fybogel
- Citrucel
- Fibercon

Most are widely available at drug stores and pharmacies and don't require a prescription (they are not drugs, just a dietary supplement). These supplements are available as powders that you mix with water and drink, or as caplets that are either chewable or meant to be swallowed whole with a glass of water.

If you're at all prone to bloating or gas please avoid both psyllium and inulin found in Metamucil, Konsyl, Fybogel, Fibersure, and FiberChoice, which can seriously worsen these problems in some people with IBS. Also, be aware that the sugar-free versions of the soluble fibre supplements can contain artificial sweeteners, which can trigger diarrhoea, gas, and cramps.

If you have gas or bloating from taking a supplement that doesn't disappear after a week or so, don't be discouraged, just try a different brand and perhaps a different formula (the pills instead of powder, or vice versa). It may take several different tries to find the soluble fibre supplement that works best for you, but the results will be well worth the effort. It's also crucial that you start at a low dose and increase gradually, to give your gut time to adjust to the fibre increase.

> NOTE: Soluble fibre supplements are often marketed as laxatives - they are **NOT**. They will **relieve** and **prevent** constipation and they are just as **effective** at treating diarrhoea **will not compromise** normal bowel function once your IBS is under control - they'll simply keep things **normal**.

THE WRONG FOODS TO EAT

While there are a variety of foods that you can eat that won't trigger an episode of IBS, there are also many foods that you should avoid. These foods may trigger bloating and gas. Foods such as:

- Dairy products (people who experience symptoms after eating dairy products should avoid milk, soft cheese, ice cream, frozen yogurt, and other dairy-based foods)
- Carbonated beverages
- Raw fruits (fructose-containing foods such as grapes, dates, bananas, raisins, honey, and figs)
- Nuts
- Cruciferous vegetables such as broccoli, cauliflower, cabbage, and Brussels sprouts
- Wheat and other gluten-containing foods prompt symptoms
- Eating high-fat, greasy foods can stimulate colonic contractions, you may do better eating smaller meals that are low in fat

- Caffeine (coffee, tea, chocolate and cola drinks), alcohol (beer, wine and "mixed" drinks) and foods that are known to produce symptoms
- Coleslaw
- Baked beans
- Items containing sorbitol (sugar-free gums, apple juice, grape juice and pear juice)
- Low-fat bakery products
- Smokers should beware: IBS symptoms may be aggravated by nicotine
- Antacids that contain magnesium

> *NOTE:* Because dairy products are an **important source** of calcium and other nutrients that your body needs, be sure to get adequate nutrients in the foods that you substitute. In addition, if milk and other dairy products bother you, you may be "lactose intolerant", which means that your body can't digest the sugar, or lactose, in milk. Dietary supplements are available to aid in digesting milk and milk products for lactose intolerant people

For gassy foods such as beans, lentils, and many vegetables, there is Beano, a brand-name digestive enzyme. Beano contains the sugar-digesting enzyme that the body needs (and which some people lack) to digest the complex sugar raffinose. If you have trouble digesting raffinose the sugar will ferment in your colon, producing gas and intestinal distress. Beano breaks down raffinose into simple sugars that cause no GI discomfort. Beano is available at health food stores in either tablets or drops, and is simply taken at the beginning of a meal. There are no side effects unless you have a rare sensitivity or allergy, and the product can be used every day.

It is important to remember that many kinds of food and drink appear to play a key role in triggering IBS attacks. Foods and drinks that healthy people can ingest without any trouble may be disruptive to IBS patients, which probably explain why IBS attacks often occur shortly after meals.

The pattern of what can and cannot be tolerated is different for each person. No two IBS patients are alike. One size does not fit all here. Because of our **"human"** uniqueness, foods ingested will react differently in each IBS patient. In addition, characteristically, IBS symptoms rarely occur at night and disrupt sleep.

CHANGES FOR IBS SUFFERERS

There is **no** single diet for IBS sufferers as IBS is an individual condition and foods react differently in IBS sufferers. Therefore, it must be treated on an individual basis. One change that may work for you, may not work for other sufferers. However, it is important to add this information to help in understanding the role of food and IBS and to give you general ideas and suggestions to assist you in managing your IBS.

I think that you can make your own diet plan based on the right foods to eat list found in this book and based on the many recipes you will find here as well. Also, use the severity levels of IBS listed next to help you determine which approach of diet and some medications based on your level of symptoms is best in helping you to make changes needed.

Mild symptoms

If you experience mild symptoms of IBS, it is recommended that you eat a ***low-fat, high-fibre diet***. Problem-causing substances should be avoided such as:

- Lactose
- Caffeine
- Beans
- Cabbage
- Cucumbers
- Broccoli
- Fatty foods
- Alcohol
- Medications

Bran or 15–25 grams a day of over-the-counter psyllium (Metamucil or Fiberall) may help both constipation and diarrhoea and are encouraged. You can still have milk or milk products if lactose intolerance is not a problem and people with irregular bowel habits, particularly constipated people, may be helped by establishing set times for meals and bathroom visits.

Moderate symptoms

The advice given above for mild cases applies here as well. Although a high-fibre diet remains the standard treatment for constipated people and laxatives such as lactulose or sorbitol may be prescribed and Imodium or Questran are suggested for diarrhoea. Abdominal pain after meals can be reduced by taking:

- Anaspaz
- Cystospaz
- Levsin
- Bemote
- Bentyl
- or Di-Spaz before eating

Psychological counselling or behavioural therapy is also suggested for some people to reduce anxiety and to learn to cope with the pain and other symptoms of IBS. Relaxation therapy, hypnosis, yoga, biofeedback, and cognitive-behavioural therapy are various types of behavioural therapy.

Severe symptoms

Again, the advice given above for mild cases applies here as well. When IBS produces constant pain that interferes with everyday life, anti-depressant drugs can help by blocking pain transmission from the nervous system. It is also important to have an ongoing and supportive doctor-patient relationship.

Alternative treatment

There has been a tendency to turn to alternative therapies in the treatment of IBS where standard therapies have not been totally successful. As a result, more dietary supplements, vitamins and herbal preparations have been utilized by IBS patients than in non-IBS patients.

Alternative and mainstream approaches to IBS treatment overlap to a certain extent. Like mainstream doctors, alternative practitioners advise a ***high-fibre diet*** as well to reduce digestive system irritation. They also suggest avoiding all of the dietary items mentioned above. Recommended stress management techniques such as reflexology may be helpful with IBS symptoms. Reflexology is a technique of foot massage that is thought to relieve diarrhoea, constipation, and other IBS symptoms.

Alternative treatments also emphasize herbal supplements such as:

- Ginger
- Buckthorn
- Enteric-coated peppermint oil

Enteric coating prevents digestion until the peppermint oil reaches the small intestine, thus avoiding irritation of the upper part of the digestive tract. Peppermint oil has been a traditional remedy for functional bowel disorders and is an ingredient in many over-the-counter remedies for the symptoms of IBS In addition; Chamomile, Valerian, Rosemary, Lemon balm and other herbs are recommended for their anti-spasmodic properties.

As a matter of fact, the list of ***alternative treatments*** for IBS is in fact quite long. It includes:

- Aromatherapy
- Homeopathy
- Hydrotherapy
- Juice therapy
- Acupuncture

- Chiropractic
- Osteopathy
- Naturopathic medicine
- Traditional Chinese herbal medicine (Chinese herbal medicine has been used for centuries in China for a variety of gastrointestinal conditions)

EATING PLAN FOR PEOPLE WITH IBS

As I stated earlier, there is no one diet that will fit all IBS sufferers. However, the following suggestions can be used to formulate your own IBS eating plan. Try variations and through the process of elimination, you will find a plan that is best suited for you.

- Eat a varied diet and avoid foods high in fat
- Drink plenty of water
- Try eating 6 small meals a day rather than 3 larger ones
- Use soy or rice replacements for dairy
- Use two egg whites to replace a whole egg
- Try low-fat vegetarian versions of meat products
- Replace some oil with fruit purees in breads or cakes
- Use veggie broth instead of oil in sauces
- Bake with cocoa powder instead of solid chocolate
- Use herbs and baking extracts (vanilla, peppermint, maple, etc.)
- Use mild spices generously to heighten flavours

Now, you'll be ready to go shopping, re-stock the pantry with your new safe staples and learn how to cook fast, easy, fabulous meals.

NOTE: If you're currently trying to **break the cycle** of ongoing attacks, it is best to strictly limit your diet to soluble fibre foods and peppermint tea for several days. This will allow your GI tract to stabilize and then you can gradually add in other foods.

A typical meal plan for IBS sufferers

This meal plan is to be used as a guideline only. It provides 25 - 30 g of fibre from a variety of sources and 30 - 35 g of fat depending on the quantity of added margarine, oil and fat content of dairy foods.

Breakfast - a bowl of high fibre cereal such as un-toasted muesli, weetabix or porridge with fresh fruit and reduced fat milk or calcium-fortified soymilk. Whole meal or grain toast with minimal margarine and honey or marmite.

Lunch - sandwiches made with whole meal bread with low fat cheese, lean beef, tinned fish and salad. Fresh fruit with low fat yoghurt. Water, tea or diluted juice.

Main Meal - water, lean grilled chicken with lemon juice and pepper, served with salad, boiled new potatoes and whole meal bread.

Snacks- spread throughout the day - fresh fruit, low fat yoghurt, crackers with cheese, or whole meal crumpets with honey. Water, tea or diluted juice.

The next section goes into more detail about typical sample meals to give you more variety. The above sample was created to give you a basic idea of what you should consider as part of your daily meal plan.

Additionally, delicious recipes for you to incorporate into your IBS meal plan follow in the recipe section.

CHAPTER 8

IBS DIET MENU

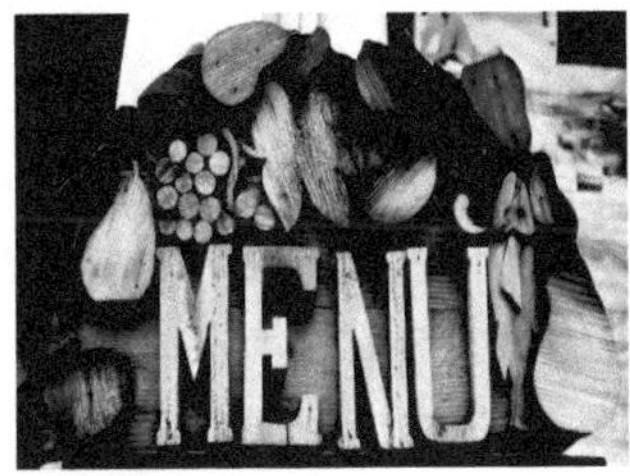

This is a sample of a day's eating on an **IBS diet**, (for illustrative purposes only) to give you options to eat a variety of possible foods. As said earlier, no one diet works for all IBS sufferers, it is a matter of personal trial and error to see what works and avoid what isn't working.

Breakfast

1-cup soy yoghurt

2 tbsp sugar-free granola or 1 cup oatmeal w/. Strawberries

1/2-cup fruit smoothie (soy/rice milk and fruit)

Mid-Morning Snack

2 oatcakes or 1 slice oat bread with light margarine, or 1 apple

Lunch Option 1

1-cup lentil soup

1 whole-wheat 6" pita

1 oz hummus

2 cups mixed salad leaves

2 tbsp fat-free dressing

Lunch

3 egg whites

1 chopped bell pepper

1/2-cup spinach

2 slices French/sourdough bread

Mid Afternoon Snack

1/2 cup unsweetened apple juice

1 mashed banana or 2 rye crackers, or handful dried apricots

Dinner

6" tortilla

5 oz turkey breast cut in thin strips

2 tsp olive oil

1 cup sliced bell peppers

1-cup spinach

1/2-cup vegetable juice

Dinner Option 2

1/2-cup mango juice or apple juice

4oz any fish grilled

1/2 cup mashed parsnips and carrots

1/2 cup boiled potatoes or cooked rice, or soba noodles

Dessert

Stewed apple with soy yogurt, or

1-cup fruit smoothie (soy/rice milk and fruit)

Substitution, Not Deprivation

Substitute soy, rice, or oat milk for all dairy milk (check the ingredients to be sure there is no oil added). Try a wide variety of brands and flavours, as the difference in taste can be dramatic. Some brands are truly horrid and some are delicious.

Meal Plan Tips

The following are additional tips that you can use to help you create your IBS meal plan.

- Keep two types of soy or rice milk on hand: unsweetened or plain for cooking and vanilla for cold cereals or drinking. Chocolate soy milk is delicious cold and heated up for glass of hot cocoa as well

- Use low-fat soy or rice substitutes for cheese, cream cheese, sour cream, ice cream, yogurt and other dairy products. For cheese, pay attention to whether the brand is truly dairy-free or simply lactose-free
- Many hamburger-based recipes such as tacos, sloppy Joes, chili, etc. can be easily adapted to IBS meal plans by substituting hamburger for TVP (textured vegetable protein, a soy food available in health food stores). Eliminate the cooking oil and season the TVP as you would the meat. When well-prepared most people honestly can't taste the difference
- Find a well-stocked local health food store and try a wide variety of vegan versions of deli meat, hot dogs, burgers, chicken wings, etc. There are tasty versions of just about every fast food and junk food on the market - just check the ingredients for a low fat content
- Use only fat-free salad dressings, mayonnaise, etc.
- Substitute cocoa powder for solid chocolate in baking
- For most recipes, you can almost always reduce the amount of oil called for by at least 1/3
- When baking replace from 2/3 to 3/4 of the oil called for with applesauce.
- Use only egg whites - simply replace each whole egg in a recipe with two egg whites. Egg Beaters are also a good choice
- Use non-stick pans and cooking spray, as this will dramatically lessen the amount of oil you cook with
- Watch out for hidden fat in seemingly safe foods: biscuits, scones, pancakes, waffles, restaurant French toast, crackers, mashed potatoes, store-bought dried (usually fried) bananas
- Eat soluble fibre first whenever your stomach is empty
- Chew thoroughly. This will help prevent you from eating too fast and swallowing air, which can cause problems
- Eat at a leisurely pace - if you must eat in a hurry, serve yourself half portions
- Eat small portions of food, and eat frequently - the emptier your stomach is, the more sensitive you will be

- Avoid eating large amounts of food in one sitting as this can trigger an attack
- Avoid ice-cold foods and drinks on an empty stomach. Cold makes muscles contract and your goal is to keep your stomach and the rest of your GI tract as calm as possible
- Avoid chewing gum, as it causes you to swallow excess air, which can trigger problems
- Drink fresh water constantly throughout the day (not ice cold). Limit the amount of water or other fluids you drink with your meals, as this can inhibit digestion
- Only eat green salads with tiny portions of non-fat dressing at the end of the meal, not the beginning
- Peel, skin, chop and cook fruits and vegetables
- Mash or puree beans, corn, peas, and berries
- Finely chop nuts, raisins and other dried fruits and fresh herbs. Nuts in particular can be quite tolerable when finely ground.

NOTE: Most soy cheese brands contain small amounts of **casein**, a dairy protein. The tiny quantity is often very tolerable for IBS, but if you're completely intolerant to **casein** you'll have to find a soy or rice cheese that is entirely dairy-free.

CHAPTER 9

HEALTHY RECIPES

MAIN DISHES

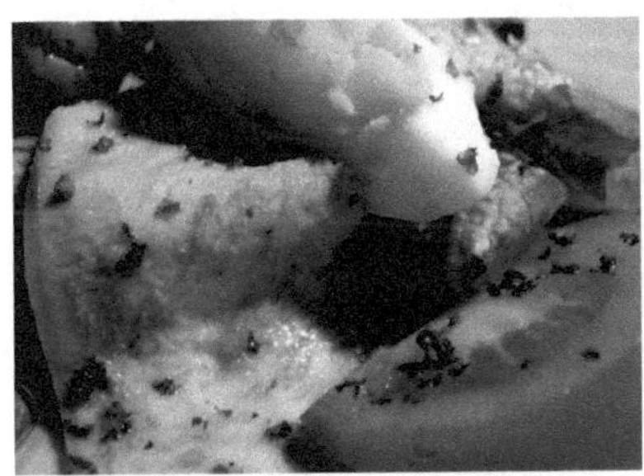

Linguine with Creamy Mushroom, Spinach, & Sherry Sauce

(Makes 6 Servings)

This pasta is elegantly rich yet hearty. If you thought you could never enjoy a luscious cream sauce again this recipe will prove you deliciously wrong. The high soluble fibre content from the linguine and French bread allow for the healthy addition of insoluble fibre from whole-wheat pastry flour and spinach - without any risk.

Ingredients

16 oz. dried linguine

4 Tablespoons olive oil

2 medium onions, diced

8 Cups mixed wild mushrooms, cleaned, and chopped

6 Tablespoons whole wheat pastry flour

2 2/3 Cups unsweetened soy or rice milk

2 Teaspoons whole grain mustard

2 Teaspoons dried marjoram

1 Cup cream sherry

1 Cup packed spinach leaves, washed, stems removed, finely shredded

salt and pepper to taste

Fresh crusty French bread for serving

Instructions

Cook the linguine in boiling salted water until tender, and drain, reserving 1/2 Cup cooking water. Heat oil in a large deep skillet and sauté onion until soft. Add the mushrooms and cook until they soften and their liquid starts to evaporate. Sift the flour into the pan and then gradually add the milk, stirring constantly until thickened and boiling. Lower heat and simmer, and add spinach, mustard, marjoram, and sherry. Cook over low heat until spinach wilts and is incorporated into sauce. Add the cooked linguine to the sauce in the skillet, and toss well to coat, adding reserved pasta cooking water if sauce is too thick. Add salt and pepper to taste. Serve immediately with crusty French bread.

New England Clam Chowder

(Makes 6 Servings)

This recipe is different than the traditional cream-based recipe. Use the easy substitution of soy or rice milk for dairy and the soup becomes perfectly safe for IBS sufferers, not to mention simply delicious.

Ingredients

1 Tablespoon olive oil

1 large onion, diced

2 large carrots, scraped and diced

1/2 Cup flour

2 Cups clam broth

3 Cups plain soy or rice milk

2 6.5 oz. cans chopped or minced clams

1/2 Teaspoon white pepper

1 Tablespoon dried parsley

3/4 Teaspoon salt

1/2 Teaspoon crushed thyme

1 bay leaf

1/4 Teaspoon ground black pepper

4 Cups baking potatoes, peeled and diced into 1 inch cubes
salt and pepper to taste for serving
fat-free Saltines crackers for serving

Instructions

In a large stockpot heat the oil over medium heat. Add the onions and carrots and sauté until softened. Gradually sift in the flour, stirring thoroughly and scraping bottom of pan. Very gradually stir in the clam broth, scraping sides and bottom of pan to make sure flour is thoroughly incorporated without clumping. Stir in rice milk until mixture is smooth. Add the clams and spices, bring soup to a boil, then cover and reduce heat. Simmer for 30 minutes. Add diced potatoes, cover and simmer for an additional 30 minutes. Taste and adjust seasoning with salt and pepper. Serve with crushed Saltines.

Chablis Chicken

(Makes 6 Servings)

Another traditional recipe, this chicken recipe didn't need a single modification for the IBS kitchen. It's perfectly safe and utterly delicious just the way it is.

Ingredients

3 whole organic chicken breasts, skinless & boneless
1/2 teaspoon salt
1/4 teaspoon freshly ground black pepper
2 tablespoons canola oil
1 cup Chablis wine
1/2 cup apple jelly
1/2 cup currants, diced
cooked rice for serving

Instructions

Sprinkle chicken with salt and pepper and set aside. In a large non-stick skillet heat oil over medium heat and cook chicken until golden brown, about four minutes per side. Remove chicken from skillet. Add to skillet Chablis, apple jelly, and currants, and simmer, stirring constantly, until bubbly and smooth.

Return chicken to skillet and baste with sauce. Cover pan and simmer 20-30 minutes or until chicken is just cooked through. Serve with rice.

Italian Crostini with Honey-Tomato Sauce & Saffron Prawns

(Makes 3-4 Servings)

This recipe has a fabulous combination of flavours - toasty fresh bread, subtly sweet and cumin-scented tomato sauce, and intensely saffron-flavoured prawns. The colours of this dish are beautiful as well the saffron tints the prawns a brilliant yellow against the scarlet sauce. The longer you simmer the tomatoes the better - the liquid will reduce and the flavours will mellow and richen. Leftover sauce and prawns are easily frozen, and very handy to have in the freezer for a 5-minute dinner.

Ingredients

For Prawns

1 cup water

6 large garlic cloves, minced

dash salt

1/8 teaspoon saffron threads

1 lb. medium prawns, shelled and de-veined

Instructions

Bring water to boil in small saucepan with garlic, salt, and saffron. Add prawns and simmer just until pink and curled. Reserve 1/4 c. cooking liquid and drain prawns. Slice each prawn in half lengthwise.

Ingredients

For Sauce

3 large ripe tomatoes, diced

1 small onion, diced

3 large cloves garlic, minced

1 1/2 tablespoons honey

1 teaspoon olive oil

1/4 teaspoon ground cumin

1/8 teaspoon cayenne pepper, or to taste

1/4 cup reserved prawn cooking liquid

Instructions

Combine all sauce ingredients in medium saucepan. Bring to a boil, reduce heat and simmer about 45 minutes, until thickened. Puree the sauce in a blender.

Ingredients

For Crostini

French or Sourdough bread baguette, sliced into 1 inch slices

2 tablespoons soy Parmesan cheese

Instructions

Place bread slices on cookie sheet and broil until golden. Turn slices over and broil other side. Top with the saffron sauce, prawn halves, and a light sprinkle of soy Parmesan. Return to broiler until cheese slightly melts. Serve immediately.

Crispy Pizza with Chicken, Scallions, & Barbecue Sauce

(Makes Two-16 inch pizzas, 8 slices per pizza)

This is a delicious, fast, and easy pizza that kids as well as adults will love.

Ingredients

Pizza Dough

1 1/2 cup warm water (105-115F)

1-tablespoon active dry yeast

4 cups all-purpose unbleached white flour

2 teaspoons salt

Instructions

In a small bowl stir together water and yeast until yeast dissolves. In a large bowl whisk together flour and salt and add yeast liquid, stirring with a wooden spoon until a soft dough forms. Knead dough until smooth and elastic, about 10 minutes, on a lightly floured surface.

Spray a large bowl lightly with cooking oil and transfer dough to bowl. Cover with plastic wrap and a kitchen towel, and let dough rise in a warm, draft-free place until doubled in bulk, about 1 1/2 hours.

Punch down dough and cut into two pieces, then form each piece into a ball. Put each ball of dough into a separate, lightly oiled large bowl and cover each bowl with a kitchen towel. Place bowls in a warm draft-free place, and let dough rise until again doubled in bulk, about 1 hour. Roll out each ball of dough separately into a 16-inch circle and transfer dough to pizza pans or stones.

Ingredients

Topping

2/3-cup Smoky Sweet Barbecue Sauce (or fat-free bottled sauce)

1 cup cooked shredded skinless organic chicken breasts

1/4 cup finely diced scallions

Ingredients

Smoky Sweet Barbecue Sauce

12-14 oz. ketchup

1/2 cup white vinegar

1/4 cup honey

1/2 - 1 teaspoon ground chipotle, to taste

1/8 teaspoon salt

Instructions

(Makes about 1 1/2 cups sauce)

Combine all ingredients in a small saucepan and simmer stirring frequently until reduced, about 15-20 minutes. Preheat oven to 450F. Brush dough very lightly with olive oil. Bake un-topped dough for 5-7 minutes or until it is dry but not browning. Remove from oven, spread evenly with barbecue sauce and sprinkle with chicken and scallions.

Bake for another 5-7 minutes or until edges are crispy and lightly browned.

Salmon Fish Cakes
(Makes 4 servings)

Ingredients

1 1/2 cups cold mashed potatoes

1 (14 ounce) can salmon (organic preferred)

1 tablespoon unsalted butter, melted, if potato does not have enough, plus extra unsalted butter, for frying

1 pinch cayenne

1/2 grated lemon, zest of

Salt and pepper to taste

1/2-cup matzo meal

2 eggs

Instructions

In large bowl mix together all fish ingredients with hands. Cover sheet with plastic wrap. Plunge hands back into mixture and form fat palm size patties. Place on sheet. Put in fridge for 20 min to 1hr. Coating mix: In shallow bowl beat 2 eggs. Dip fish in egg then in 1/2 cup Matzo meal. Coat well. Melt butter and a bit of oil and fry till golden brown. About 4-6 min each side.

CHAPTER 10

DESERTS

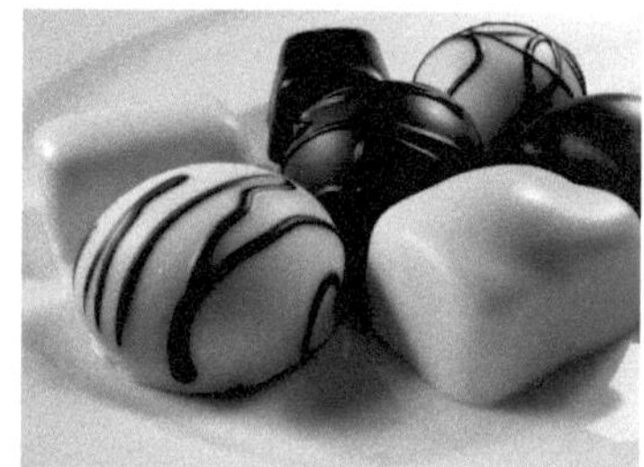

Peppermint Fudge Cake

(Makes 12 Servings)

This recipe is sinfully rich with deep dark chocolate, ridiculously easy to make, and completely delicious.

Ingredients

Sift together in large bowl and whisk together well:

1 level Tablespoon Acacia Tummy Fibre (optional)

2 Cups all-purpose flour

2 Teaspoons baking soda

6 Tablespoons unsweetened cocoa powder

1 Tablespoon cornstarch

1 Cup white sugar

1/2 Teaspoon salt

Whisk together by hand in medium bowl:

1 3/4 Cup unsweetened applesauce

1/4 Cup canola oil

1 Tablespoon vanilla

1 Tablespoon peppermint extract

Instructions

Preheat oven to 325F.

Spray a 10-inch bundt pan with cooking oil and set aside. Add the wet ingredients to the dry with a few swift strokes just until blended. Pour into bundt pan. Bake 50-60 minutes, until a toothpick comes out with moist crumbs. Cool on rack.

Double Decker Sweet Potato Pecan Pie

(Makes 8 servings)

Raise oven temperature to 350F. In a large bowl mix all ingredients until well blended and completely smooth. Set aside.

Ingredients

Pecan Filling

6 organic egg whites

1/2 Cup granulated sugar

1/2 Teaspoon salt

2 Tablespoons canola oil

1 1/2 Cups light corn syrup

1 Cup finely chopped fresh pecan halves

1 Tablespoon vanilla extract

Instructions

Combine first 5 ingredients in large bowl and beat thoroughly until well combined. Stir in pecans and vanilla. Pour sweet potato filling into baked pie crust and smooth top. Carefully pour pecan filling on top. Bake for 1 hour to 1 hour 15 minutes, until a knife inserted into the pie comes out clean. Cool on rack.

Banana Butterscotch Soufflés

(Makes 4 Servings)

The soufflés rise high and golden above their bowls, and inside they are creamy, sweet, and rich. They're almost fat free and full of soluble fibre.

Ingredients

3 large organic egg whites

1/4 cup granulated sugar

2 firm-ripe bananas

2 tablespoons butterscotch chips, finely chopped

Instructions

Preheat oven to 450F and spray four 2-cup capacity ramekins or bowls with cooking oil. In a large bowl beat egg whites until they hold soft peaks and gradually beat in sugar until egg whites hold stiff peaks. Coarsely grate the bananas into the meringue and fold in with the butterscotch chips.

Place ramekins on a cookie sheet and fill with batter, mounding it in centers and running a knife along the sides of ramekins to aid rising. Bake in center of oven for 15 minutes, or until puffed and golden brown. Serve immediately (soufflés will deflate quickly).

Sweet Cherry Almond Cake

(Makes 14-16 Servings)

This recipe is fast, easy, low fat, packed with soluble fibre, and has the added goodness of fresh fruit and almonds. It's even low in sugar for a dessert. Most importantly, it's absolutely delicious.

Ingredients

3/4 cup almonds, finely ground

1/2 cup packed brown sugar

1/3 cup plus 3 tablespoons unbleached white flour

6 large organic egg whites

1/4 teaspoon salt

1/4 cup canola oil

1 1/2 teaspoons vanilla

1 1/2 teaspoons almond extract

2 cups cooked cherries*

1/2 teaspoon granulated sugar

Instructions

*To cook fresh cherries, pit them and place in a small saucepan with 1 T.

water. Bring to a boil and reduce heat, simmering just until cherries soften and cook down, but haven't disintegrated.

Preheat oven to 375F. Spray a 10-inch non-stick spring form pan with cooking oil and set aside. In a medium bowl whisk together almonds, brown sugar, and flour until well combined. In a large bowl beat egg whites with salt until they just hold stiff peaks and fold in nut mixture gently but thoroughly. Fold in oil, vanilla, and almond extract, and spread batter in prepared pan.
Arrange cherries evenly over batter and sprinkle with granulated sugar. Bake cake for 20-30 minutes or until a tester comes out clean. Cool on rack.

Will's Dreamy Lemon Rice Pudding

(Makes 6 Servings)

This is unlike any rice pudding you've ever had before. It is so light and creamy it's practically a mousse. It is the perfect food for IBS, full of soluble fibre and with almost zero fat. It's terrific for helping to stabilize your digestion and break an ongoing cycle of IBS attacks.

Ingredients

1/4 cup Acacia Tummy Fibre
3 cups soy milk (rice milk will not give as creamy results)
3 cups water
1/4-teaspoon salt
1/2-teaspoon canola oil
1/4 cup granulated sugar
5 organic egg whites, whipped until they just barely hold soft peaks
3 cups cold cooked short grain white rice, such as calrose or sushi rice
Zest of 1 lemon, grated or minced (do NOT use lemon juice)
1 teaspoon vanilla
2 tablespoons chopped raisins (optional)

Instructions

Add the Acacia to a small bowl, and whisk in just enough of the soy milk to dissolve the Acacia. In a large stockpot, over medium heat, bring soymilk and Acacia mixture, remaining soy milk, and water just barely to a boil. Because the whipped egg whites in the recipe rise significantly as they cook, it is essential that you use a large stockpot or the pudding will boil over. With a metal whisk add in the salt, oil, and sugar.

While whisking constantly, add several very large spoonfuls of hot milk into the egg whites to temper (blend without scrambling) the eggs. Add the tempered egg whites to the saucepan of milk and whisk thoroughly, cooking for 2-3 minutes.

Add rice and cook, whisking frequently without scraping the bottom of the pan, until mixture thickens slightly, about 20-30 minutes (pudding will thicken further as it cools). Remove from heat and add zest, vanilla, and raisins. Serve warm or chill.

Chocolate Silk Pudding

(Makes 6 Servings)

This recipe makes what is undoubtedly the richest pudding (it is hard to believe that it is virtually fat-free).

Ingredients

3 level tablespoons Acacia Tummy Fibre (optional)

6 tablespoons granulated sugar

1/2 cup unsweetened cocoa powder

6 tablespoons cornstarch

dash salt

3 organic egg whites

3 cups vanilla soy/rice milk

6 tablespoons dark corn syrup

1 tablespoon vanilla extract

1/2 teaspoon almond extract (optional)

Instructions

In a heavy, large double boiler whisk together all ingredients to salt. In a small bowl beat the egg whites until lightly frothy. Set eggs aside. Gradually whisk into the double boiler the milk and corn syrup, and scrape around the bottom and edges of the pan with a rubber spatula until thoroughly blended. Set pan over boiling water and cook, whisking constantly until the mixture reaches a full boil. Continue whisking for one more minute, and remove from heat.

Carefully whisk several large spoonfuls of hot pudding into the egg whites to temper them. Add the egg mixture back to the pan of pudding and whisk well to thoroughly blend. Return the pan to the heat and whisk constantly for one minute until mixture thickens. Remove from heat and whisk in vanilla (and almond) extract. Pour into six serving glasses and chill until cold. Variations: Pudding may also be used as pie filling with a graham cracker crust, or frozen in an ice cream maker according to manufacturer's directions.

CHAPTER 11

BEVERAGES

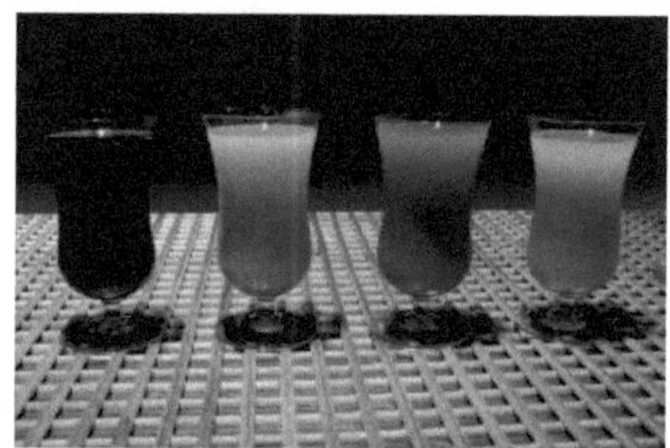

High-Energy Banana Carob Breakfast Shake

(Makes 1 serving, easily doubled or tripled)

Breakfast in a glass! Fast, easy, and nutritious, this drink is a great start to any day. It's low in fat and in high soluble fibre.

Ingredients

1 firm-ripe banana

1 organic egg white (If salmonella is a concern in your area you can substitute pasteurized egg whites, available in the dairy section of most grocery stores (Egg Beaters, etc.)

1/4-cup vanilla soy or rice milk

2 tablespoons carob powder

Instructions

Combine all ingredients in blender and puree until smooth, scraping down sides of blender with rubber spatula if necessary. Pour into a large glass and serve.

Virgin Strawberry Daiquiris

(Makes 4 Servings)

These daiquiris are summer in a glass – ruby-red, sweet, and luscious. Blending the berries makes their insoluble fibre much more tolerable. For guests who prefer their drinks sinful to virginal, add spiced rum to the daiquiris to taste. Serve this drink with a meal.

Ingredients

1/2 cup Rose's lime juice

1/4 - 1/3 cup granulated sugar

juice of half an orange

4 cups frozen fresh whole strawberries, very slightly thawed

Instructions

Combine all ingredients except the strawberries in a blender and blend well. Slowly add the strawberries a few at a time and blend well after each addition. Pour into glasses and serve immediately with a meal.

Soothing Sweet Peppermint Green Tea

(Makes 6 Servings)

Great breakfast tea, especially for cold winter mornings.

Ingredients

2 Cups packed fresh mint leaves

1/2 Cup sugar

6 Cups boiling water

1 1/2 Teaspoons green tea powder

Instructions

Place all ingredients but tea powder in a teapot, and stir to dissolve the sugar. Let steep 4 minutes, add the tea powder, and let steep 1 minute. Stir well. Serve hot or chilled.

Mexican Cinnamon-Lime Horchatas

(Makes 4 Servings)

A **horchata** is a Mexican iced drink made from groundnuts, seeds, or rice. The high soluble fibre content of almonds makes this a safe drink, particularly because the nuts are so finely ground. This recipe is smooth, light, and refreshing, and offers a delicious accompaniment to many foods. For a sweet and soothing end to a hot summer day, pour a glass to enjoy after dinner as you sit on your front porch and watch the sun go down. If you wish to double this recipe, make two separate batches or you will overfill your blender.

Ingredients

1 Cup sliced almonds

2 Cup boiling water

1 large cinnamon stick, broken into pieces

grated zest from one lime

1/2 Cup granulated sugar

2 Cups crushed ice cubes

Instructions

In a blender combine all ingredients except ice. Let sit for 15-minutes. Blend mixture on high speed for 3-4 minutes. Add ice and blend for 2 minutes. Slowly pour mixture into a large pitcher through a fine mesh sieve or a double layer of dampened cheese cloth, pressing hard on solids to extract as much liquid as possible. Discard solids. Chill the filled pitcher until cold, and preferably overnight. Pour into ice-filled glasses.

CHAPTER 12

SNACKS / APPETIZERS

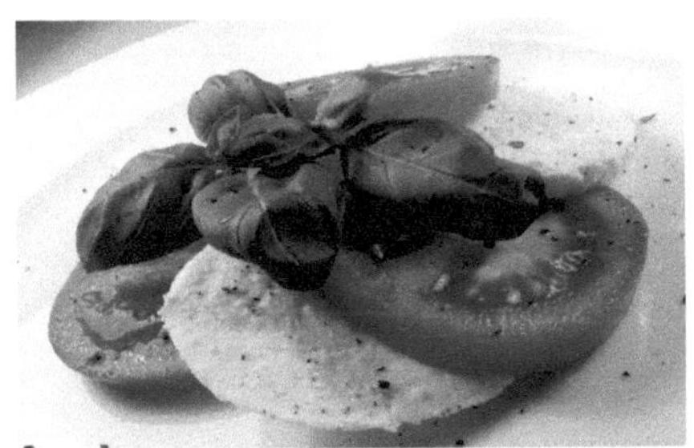

Honey Glazed Snack Mix

(Makes 10 Half-cup Servings)

This mix is crunchy, sweet, and salty all at once, and is a delicious way to stabilize if you're in the midst of a cycle of attacks. Keep bags at work for the afternoon munchies. It's also great snack food for road trips.

Ingredients

3 tablespoons canola oil

1/4 cup honey

2 cups Corn Chex cereal

2 cups Rice Chex cereal

1 cup mini pretzels

Instructions

In a small bowl stir together oil and honey until well blended. In a large bowl stir together cereals and pretzels, top with honey mixture, and stir until well combined. Microwave on high for 5-6 minutes, stirring well every 90 seconds until cooked through. Cool thoroughly before serving.

Sweet Mango and Roasted Tomato Salsa

(Makes 6 Servings)

This recipe is a great example of how spices can be perfectly safe even when they're a little hot - the key is the soluble fibre base from the baked corn chips.

Ingredients

5 ripe plum tomatoes

1 teaspoon ground chipotle pepper, or to taste*

1/4 cup fresh lime juice

2 tablespoons honey

2 small ripe mangoes, peeled and diced

baked corn chips (Tostitos) for serving

Instructions

Roast or broil tomatoes until skin blisters and blackens, turning to cook evenly on all sides. Add tomatoes, chipotle, lime, and honey to a blender and puree until smooth. Pour into serving bowl and stir in diced mango. Adjust ratio of limejuice or honey to taste. Serve with baked corn chips.

Portabella Mushroom and Sundried Tomato Bruschetta

(Makes 3-4 Servings)

This recipe is fast, easy, and delicious. It makes a great safe snack in a hurry, and the leftovers are perfect to take to work for lunch the next day.

Ingredients

1/2 cup water

1/4 cup packed dried tomatoes

1 teaspoon balsamic vinegar

2 portabella mushroom caps, cleaned and chopped (about 3/4 lb.)

2 garlic cloves, minced

1 tablespoon olive oil

2 tablespoons finely shredded fresh basil

salt and pepper to taste

Two 12 inch long sourdough bread baguettes, halved and toasted

Instructions

In a small saucepan heat the water until it boils. Remove from heat and add tomatoes; soak for 15 minutes. Puree tomatoes, cooking water, and vinegar in blender and transfer to serving bowl. In a medium non-stick skillet sprayed with cooking oil sauté the mushrooms and garlic over medium heat until tender, and the liquid released from mushrooms has evaporated (about 5 minutes). Remove from heat and stir in the olive oil. Fold mushrooms into tomato mixture and add chopped basil. Season with salt and pepper to taste. Serve with baguette.

Grilled Shrimp Shish Kebabs with Spanish Saffron Sauce

(Makes 6 Servings)

Brilliant golden yellow, smooth and creamy, the pungency of this saffron and garlic aioli sauce plays off the mellow sweetness of grilled shrimp. Shrimp are a great source of protein for an IBS diet because they are so low fat, and the dip is loaded with soluble fibre from the bread and almond base.

Ingredients

1 1/2 pound shrimp, shelled

1 Teaspoon dried rosemary

2 Tablespoon olive oil, divided

1/4 Teaspoon saffron threads

2 Cups packed, one-inch cubes of French bread, soaked 15 minutes in 1/2 Cup water

2 large garlic cloves

1/4 Cup almonds, finely ground

6 Tablespoons fresh lemon juice

1/4 Teaspoon salt

2 Tablespoons water

Instructions

In a bowl stir together the shrimp, rosemary, and 1 Tablespoon olive oil, and marinate, chilled, for 1 hour. Place saffron threads in a small saucer and microwave for 10-20 seconds, until brittle. Add saffron, remaining 1

Tablespoon olive oil, and all other ingredients to a food processor or blender, and puree until smooth, scraping down sides with a rubber spatula as necessary. Transfer dip to serving bowl. Thread shrimp on metal skewers and grill over medium high heat in grill pan (or over charcoal grill) just until cooked through, about 2 minutes per side. Serve shrimp with dipping sauce.

Smoky Eggplant Hummus

(Makes 6-8 servings)

This Lebanese-inspired dip tastes incredible. The eggplant is the secret to its silky texture, and the low overall fat content and high soluble fibre in the chickpeas (which are pureed until smooth) makes it a safe choice.

Ingredients

1 medium eggplant (about 1 pound)

1 Cup cooked or canned chickpeas, rinsed and drained

1 large garlic clove, mashed

2 Tablespoons well-stirred tahini

1/4 Teaspoon salt

1/4 Cup fresh lemon juice

1 Tablespoon finely chopped fresh flat-leaf parsley

Pita bread for serving

Instructions

Preheat broiler or prepare a grill. Prick eggplant in several places with a fork. Broil or grill about 3-4 inches from heat, turning every 10 minutes or so, until eggplant is charred all over and very soft (about 45 minutes). Put eggplant in a bowl to cool and collect juices. When cold, peel skin off eggplant, discard skin, and transfer pulp to a blender or food processor. Add all remaining ingredients except parsley and puree until very smooth, scraping down sides with a rubber spatula as necessary. Transfer to serving bowl and sprinkle with parsley. Serve with fresh pita bread.

CHAPTER 13

BREAKFAST & BREADS

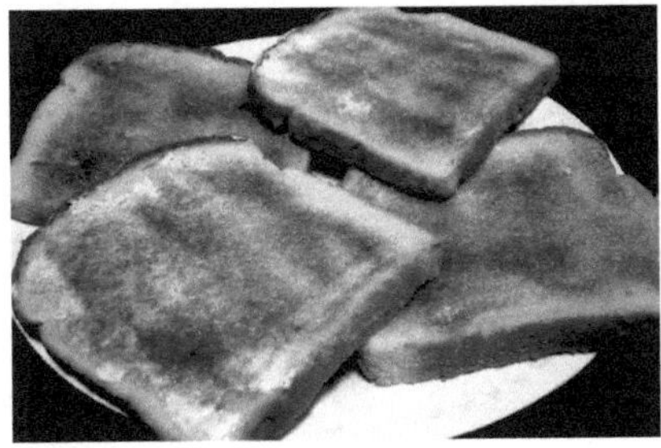

Mushroom, Crab and Dill Omelette

(Makes 1 serving, easily doubled or tripled)

Crab, and the combination of savoury sautéed mushrooms with the sweet seafood are irresistible. Using all egg whites and no yolks makes this a perfectly safe breakfast.

Ingredients

2 organic egg whites

1/4 teaspoon dill weed

2/3 cup finely chopped fresh mushrooms

1 tablespoon finely chopped fresh onion

2 tablespoons crab meat

French or sourdough toast for serving

Instructions

In a small bowl combine egg whites with dill, whisking until lightly frothy. In a small non-stick skillet sprayed with cooking oil sauté the mushrooms and onions until tender and liquid from mushrooms evaporates. Transfer mushrooms and onions to a small bowl and mix with crabmeat. Wipe clean the skillet with a paper towel, spray with cooking oil and heat over medium. Add egg mixture and immediately top with filling ingredients, forming a narrow line of filling across the center of the omelette. When edges of the omelette are slightly crisp, carefully roll omelette up from one side with a rubber spatula to completely enclose filling, turn omelette over, and cook on other side for an additional 1-2 minutes. Serve immediately with the toast.

Caramelized Vanilla Pear Pancake

(Makes 6 Servings)

Everyone with IBS knows that breakfast is the toughest meal, and traditional pancakes are major triggers due to their high dairy and fat content. This recipe lets you enjoy a delicious morning treat without the fear of consequences.

Ingredients

1 Cup soy/rice milk

1 Tablespoon apple cider vinegar

1 1/3 Cups all-purpose flour

2 Teaspoons baking powder

1 Teaspoon baking soda

1/2 Teaspoon salt

1/2 Cup brown sugar

4 Tablespoons canola oil

8 organic egg whites

2 Tablespoons vanilla extract

5 firm-ripe fresh pears

2 Tablespoons fresh lemon juice

Instructions

Preheat oven to 400F. In a small bowl stir together the soy milk and vinegar; set aside. In a large bowl sift together flour, baking powder, baking soda, salt, and 3 Tablespoons of the brown sugar. In a small bowl with an electric mixer beat well 2 Tablespoons of the canola oil, soured soy milk, egg whites, and vanilla. Whisk by hand wet ingredients into dry until just combined. Set batter aside.

Peel and core pears, and slice lengthwise into 8 wedges per pear. Stir together remaining brown sugar and lemon juice, and add pears to coat. In a large cast-iron skillet heat remaining 2 Tablespoons of oil. Arrange pears in a spiral pattern in skillet, top with any remaining sugar mixture, and cook over medium heat until just tender and sugar begins to caramelize, about 10 minutes.

Pour batter over pears and bake in oven for 15 minutes. Reduce oven temperature to 350 and bake 5-10 minutes more, until golden and firm to touch. Remove from oven, run thin knife around edge of skillet, place heat-safe plate on top of skillet, and carefully but quickly invert. Slowly lift skillet off cake. Serve immediately.

Sweet Cinnamon Zucchini Bread

(Makes two small 9 x 5 inch loaves, 12 slices per loaf, If the recipe is doubled it will make two full-size 9 x 5 inch loaves)

This bread is just slightly sweet, very moist, and so heavenly it's hard to believe that not only is it packed with zucchini and good for you, it's also very low fat and high soluble fibre, making it a safe and delicious snack any time of day.

Ingredients

Sift into a large bowl and whisk dry ingredients with a metal whisk until thoroughly blended.

3 Cups all-purpose flour
1 Teaspoon salt
1 Teaspoon soda
1 Tablespoon cinnamon
1/4 Teaspoon baking powder

In another large bowl beat well with an electric mixer:
6 organic egg whites, beaten light and foamy
1/2 Cup canola oil
1 1/2 Cups brown sugar
2 Cups grated unpeeled zucchini
2 teaspoons vanilla

Instructions

Preheat oven to 325F. Add dry ingredients to wet with a few swift strokes by hand just until well blended. Pour batter into two non-stick loaf pans sprayed with cooking oil. Bake for about 1 hour or until a toothpick inserted into the center of the loaf comes out clean. Cool on racks.

Brown Sugar Banana Bread

(Makes two 9 x 5 inch loaves, 16 slices per loaf)

This recipe is, without a doubt, the best banana bread in the world, and it makes absolutely spectacular French toast as well.

Ingredients

Sift into a large bowl and whisk dry ingredients with a metal whisk until well blended.

3 1/2 cups all-purpose unbleached white flour

1/2 teaspoon baking powder

2 teaspoons baking soda

1/2 teaspoon salt

Ingredients

In a large bowl blend with an electric mixer until creamy:

6 organic egg whites

1/3 cup canola oil

1 1/3 cup brown sugar

1 tablespoon vanilla

3 cups mashed black bananas (6-8 bananas)*

Instructions

Preheat oven to 350F. Add dry ingredients to wet and with a few swift strokes blend by hand until smooth. Pour into non-stick loaf pans sprayed with cooking oil and bake for 50-60 minutes or until a toothpick or cake tester inserted into the center of the loaf comes out clean. Cool on rack. Recipe doubles or triples easily, and extra loaves freeze well. *The bananas have to be super-ripe for this recipe. If they're not black, they're not ready.

Old-Fashioned Vanilla French Toast & Apricot Caramel Sauce

(Makes 6 Servings)

Never go without being able to eat this because of the high fat content (from dairy, egg yolks, and oil from frying), which unfailingly triggers an IBS attack. This version, however, is completely safe.

Ingredients

1/2 of a 12.5 oz. package silken tofu, drained

2 organic egg whites

1/2 cup vanilla soy/rice milk

1 tablespoon vanilla

1 narrow loaf French or sourdough bread, slightly stale, cut diagonally into 1 inch slices

Instructions

Combine first four ingredients in a blender, and blend on high speed until smooth. Pour batter into a glass pie plate. Dip slices of bread in batter, turn over, and soak for about 10 minutes. Heat a large non-stick skillet sprayed with cooking oil over medium high, add bread slices without crowding, and cook until golden brown on the bottom. Turn the slices with a rubber spatula and lightly brown the other sides. Serve immediately with Apricot Caramel Sauce.

The French toast alone is good served with maple syrup, powdered sugar, or fruit jelly, but for a truly decadent treat try making the Apricot Caramel Sauce. The toast is slightly crunchy, a little chewy, and the sweet-tart richness of the sauce is the perfect foil.

Apricot Caramel Sauce

(Makes about 2 cups syrup)

Ingredients

1 1/2 cups granulated sugar

1 cup water
6-8 fresh ripe apricots, unpeeled, pitted and diced
2 teaspoons vanilla
juice of half a lemon

Instructions

In a medium heavy saucepan combine all ingredients except lemon juice and simmer, uncovered, until apricots disintegrate (mash with a potato masher every so often to speed the process) and mixture reduces to syrup in about 1 hour. Remove from heat and add lemon juice.

CHAPTER 14

CONDIMENTS/DRESSINGS

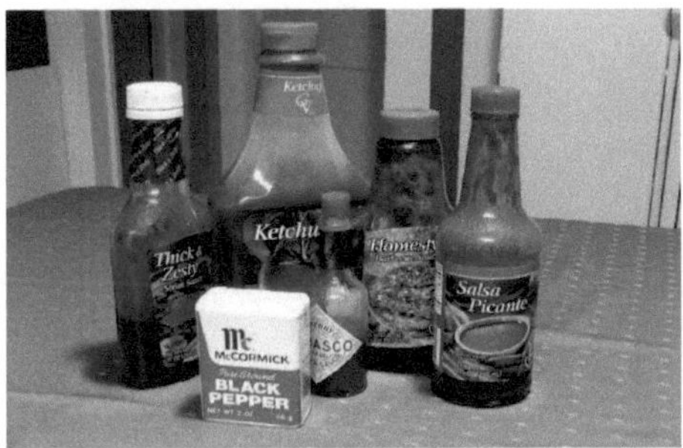

Tofu Island Dressing
(Makes 1 ½ cups)

This thick dressing is similar to Thousand Island Dressing.

Ingredients

1 (10 1/2 ounce) package lite silken tofu

1 tablespoon lemon juice

3 tablespoons ketchup or chili sauce

2 tablespoons sweet pickle relish

1 tablespoon minced parsley

1 tablespoon minced red onions

1 teaspoon soy sauce

Fresh black pepper to taste

Instructions

Place the tofu and lemon juice in blender or food processor and blend till smooth. Place in a bowl and stir in remaining ingredients. Chill for at least 2 hrs before using.

Fat Free Dijon Mustard Spread
(makes 1 ½ cups)

Ingredients

1 cup fat-free mayonnaise

1 tablespoon Dijon mustard

1 dash garlic salt

1 dash black pepper

Instructions

In a small bowl, mix all the ingredients by hand. Chill and use as needed on sandwiches, etc.

Fat Free Honey Mustard Dressing

(10 servings - 2 1/2 cups)

Ingredients

1 1/4 cups fat-free mayonnaise or fat-free Miracle Whip

1/4 cup honey

1/4 cup prepared yellow mustard

1/3 cup cider vinegar

1/4 teaspoon cayenne pepper

1/2 cup water

1 garlic clove, minced

Instructions

Place all ingredients in a bowl. Whisk or blend together.

COOKBOOKS SUITABLE FOR IBS

'Find out about fibre' by Rosemary Stanton, Allen and Unwin

'Good Gut Cookbook' by Rosemary Stanton, 2nd ed Harper Health

'Friendly Foods' by Swain, A, Soutter and Loblay, R.H, Murdoch Books

FAQ'S ON IBS

What is irritable bowel syndrome?

Irritable bowel syndrome (IBS) is a common problem with the intestines. In people with IBS, the intestines squeeze too hard or not hard enough and cause food to move too quickly or too slowly through the intestines. IBS usually begins around age 20 and is more common in women.

How is IBS treated?

The best way to handle IBS is to eat a healthy diet, avoid foods that seem to make you feel worse and find ways to handle your stress.

How is IBS diagnosed?

Your doctor may start by asking you questions about your symptoms. If your symptoms have had a pattern over time, the pattern may make it clear to your doctor that IBS is the cause.

What are the symptoms of IBS?

If your symptoms have just started, something else may be the cause. Your doctor may need to do some tests, such as a blood test or colonoscopy, to make sure that your symptoms aren't caused by something other than IBS. The symptoms may get worse when you're under stress, such as when you travel, attend social events or change your daily routine. Your symptoms may also get worse if you don't eat enough healthy foods or after you've eaten a big meal.

Do certain foods cause IBS?

No. Foods don't cause IBS. But some foods may bring on or make symptoms of IBS worse. Foods that may make symptoms worse include foods high in fat or caffeine. Fat and caffeine can cause your intestines to contract, which may cause cramping. Alcohol and chocolate may also make you feel worse.

How can stress affect IBS?

Stress may trigger symptoms in people with IBS. Talk to your family doctor about ways to deal with stress, such as exercise, relaxation training or meditation. He or she may have some suggestions or may refer you to someone who can give you some ideas. Your doctor may also suggest that you talk to a counsellor about things that are bothering you.

Will IBS get worse over time?

No. While IBS will probably recur throughout your life, it won't get worse. It doesn't cause cancer or require surgery, and it won't shorten your life.

What if IBS interferes with my daily activities?

IBS may have caused you to avoid doing certain things, like going out or going to work or school. While it may take some time for your efforts to pay off, you may find new freedom by following a plan that includes a healthy diet, learning new ways to deal with your stress and avoiding foods that may make your symptoms worse.

How long does the treatment take to relieve symptoms?

Relief of IBS Symptoms is often a slow process. It may take six months or more for definite improvement to be appreciated. Patience is extremely important in dealing with this problem.

Can IBS lead to more serious problems?

IBS does not cause cancer, bleeding or inflammatory bowel diseases, such as ulcerative colitis. Over the long term, IBS can be associated with but does not cause diverticulosis, "pockets" in the intestinal wall, which is a benign condition. Treatment of IBS with bulk agents helps to prevent diverticulosis and other colon problems.

FOOD JOURNAL SHEET

Daily Food Journal Sheet

Day: ______________________ **Date**: ______________________

Breakfast: ______________________

Mid-morning Snack: ______________________

Lunch: ______________________

Dinner: ______________________

Desert: ______________________

Notes: (note any symptoms that may have appeared from the foods eaten today). Keep this sheet as a reference to see what works and what doesn't. Discuss results with your Doctor.

CONCLUSIONS

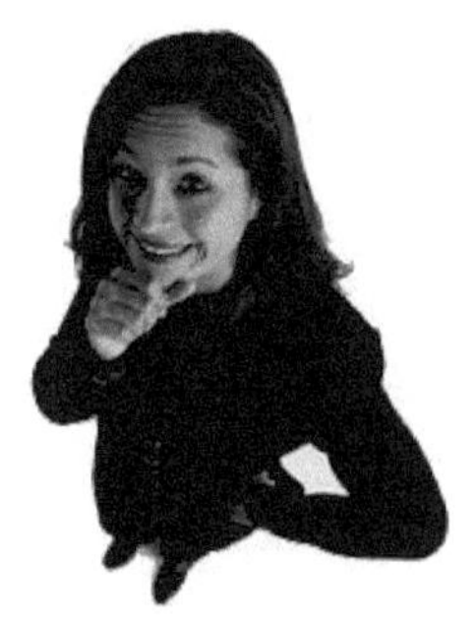

As you can see, IBS is a complex syndrome with a wide range of causes and treatments. The pathophysiology of IBS is not totally understood today. There appear to be many factors that contribute to the appearance of IBS in a patient. There are physical, mental, and hereditary characteristics that can influence the appearance of the diseasc.

There is more information available on who exactly gets IBS. We know that people within the ages of 13 to 50 are most likely to have IBS. After 50 years of age, the prevalence of the disease declines. We know that some ethnic groups have hereditary weaknesses that can cause problems similar to IBS. African-Americans, for instance, are mostly lactose-intolerant and this can contribute to the diagnosis of IBS in some cases.

To recap, IBS has a number of different potential causes that are as follows:

- Immune system irritations
- Antibiotics
- Food Sensitivities
- Allergies
- Bacterial overgrowth
- Stress
- Hormones

All of these different triggers can play a role in the development of IBS. You may actually be suffering from multiple causes. This makes treating IBS a hit or miss process. One thing that is certain, diet is a key component of any successful IBS treatment program.

It's important to recognize that IBS is a chronic syndrome that requires some dedication and perseverance to treat and overcome. It may take some time before you see some benefit and in between you may end up stressed out and depressed.
In the section on other treatments available for IBS, we discussed the types of medicines that a conventional physician might prescribe and some of their potential side effects. On top of laxatives and anti-diarrheals, we mentioned some antispasmodics, some antibiotics, and even antidepressants. All of these are part of a conventional physician's treatment options for IBS.

We gave the reader some other options when we discussed natural supplements used to treat the symptoms of IBS. These included:

- Natural fiber
- Assorted herbal remedies

In addition, we talked about the link between the use of probiotics and the establishment of good bacteria in the intestinal tract. Probiotics are becoming more and more popular with consumers and it's hoped that more foods will become available with probiotic cultures. Until then, you can get probiotics in capsule forms through distributors and natural food stores.

Finally, we arrived at the very large topic of stress relief. Strategies for stress relief rely on common sense approaches in some cases and behavior modification in others. We talked about:

- Simple and effective stress-relief strategies
- Learning how to manage your time
- Meditation
- Massage
- Exercise

Hopefully, you've gotten some practical techniques to help you deal with the stress of having IBS. Remember to keep a positive attitude and be certain that you will overcome this condition eventually.

REFERENCES AND SUPPORT LINKS FOR UK AND USA

International Foundation for Functional Gastrointestinal Disorders - USA

http://www.iffgd.org

National Digestive Diseases Information Clearinghouse - USA

http://www.digestive.niddk.nih.gov

How to Cope With Irritable Bowel Syndrome - USA
http://www.ehow.com/tips_11375.html

Eat For Wellness - USA

http://health.ivillage.com/digestion/ibs_lw/0,,jb38,00.html

Comfort Foods For Digestive Health - USA

http://comfortfoods.wordpress.com/

Patient UK - Irritable Bowel Syndrome Site for UK

http://www.patient.co.uk/showdoc/23068776/

The Gut Trust – UK

http://www.theguttrust.org/home

Net Doctor – UK

http://www.netdoctor.co.uk/diseases/facts/irritablecolon.htm

IBS Register – UK

http://www.ibsregister.com/

BBC Health Conditions – UK

http://www.bbc.co.uk/health/conditions/ibs1.shtml